Achieving Vibrance

Achieving Vibrance

A Seven-Minute-a-Day
Plan for Feeling, Looking,
and Being Younger

Gay Hendricks, Ph.D.

FOREWORD BY
Deborah Nemiro-Wilson, M.D.

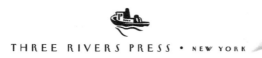

THREE RIVERS PRESS • NEW YORK

For the vibrant heart-center of my life,

KATHLYN THATCHER HENDRICKS

my wife, best friend, and creative partner.

Published by Three Rivers Press, New York, New York.

Member of the Crown Publishing Group.

Random House, Inc. New York, Toronto, London, Sydney, Auckland

www.randomhouse.com

Three Rivers Press and the Tugboat design are registered trademarks of Random House, Inc.

Printed in the United States of America

DESIGN BY LYNNE AMFT

Library of Congress Cataloging-in-Publication Data
Hendricks, Gay.
Achieving vibrance : a seven-minute-a-day plan
for feeling, looking, and being younger / by Gay Hendricks.
1. Rejuvenation.   2. Longevity.   3.Mind and body.
4. Beauty, Personal.   I. Title.
RA776.75.H46   2001
613.7—dc21   2001024806

ISBN 0-609-80939-3

10   9   8   7   6   5   4   3   2   1

First Edition

ACKNOWLEDGMENTS

I HAVE BEEN BLESSED to know many vibrant people in my life, and I would like to begin this book by thanking some of them for the remarkable wisdom they passed along to me.

My grandmother, Rebecca Delle Garrett Canaday, was the vibrant center of my family, and I give thanks every day for the blessings she gave me. She credited her long life to eating vegetables she'd grown herself, being honest in dealing with people, and spending a few minutes bending over to touch her toes every day. Although this sounded impossibly old-fashioned to me as a kid, I appreciate it more every year of my life.

Dwight Webb, Ph.D., was the first genuinely vibrant person I can recall meeting in my adult life. I studied his charismatic presence for months before I worked up the courage to ask him, "What makes you the way you are?" He said he felt vitalized in every moment because every encounter with other people was an opportunity to learn from them and love them to the best of his ability. I adopted this attitude on the spot and haven't had a dull moment since.

Jack Downing, M.D., whom I met in my mid-twenties, was that rarest of creatures: The happy adult. A quarter-century older than I, he had at least twice the energy I did. Where did his vibrance come from? Here's a hint: One day I poured out a problem to him, and he gave me a most unusual piece of advice. He recommended that I go home, turn on loud music, and dance with the problem for an hour. "That's right—dance it rather than talking about it," he said. "You're so much in your head that you get trapped going 'round in circles, trying to figure things out intellectually. Get out of your mind for an hour by moving your body to music. If everybody danced an hour a day we could close down all the mental health clinics in America."

Two of my Santa Barbara compatriots, Kenny Loggins and John Cleese, have taught me a key secret of vibrance: We only feel truly happy when we're fully committed to our creativity. Being around them has given me a benchmark question to live from: Does this (this decision, this offer, this choice) give me opportunity for full creative expression? This question has inspired me to say "No" to things as often as "Yes," and each move has grown my vibrance by leaps and bounds.

I want to thank Teresa Glenn, director of our institute, for the gift of her wit, intelligence, and enthusiasm in my life.

Acknowledgments

Hearty thanks also to Jhaura Wachsmann for his help in getting our message out to the world through our tapes and website.

I'm deeply grateful to Sandy Dijkstra, the best literary agent in the world, for her friendship, guidance, and business savvy. A deep bow of gratitude goes also to my European colleagues—Esther Staewen, Dr. Meinrad Milz, and Dr. Katrin Bieber—for their passionate commitment to conscious living and for their incredibly generous hospitality.

And finally, I'm deeply indebted to the several hundred participants in our research projects. I couldn't have done it without you, and I send you an eternity of thanks for helping us craft the exciting program that has helped so many.

CONTENTS

Contents

Deborah Nemiro-Wilson, M.D.

"I'm dog-tired."
"Why do I feel flat so often?"
"My get-up-and-go has gone and went."

AS A BUSY OBSTETRICIAN-GYNECOLOGIST, I hear these complaints week in and week out. Fatigue and lack of energy are by far the most common symptoms my patients bring to me, especially those over fifty. From a physician's standpoint, the symptoms are frustrating because 99 percent of the time there are no clear physical reasons to account for them. I have asked myself many times, "Why is this perfectly healthy person not feeling energetic and alive?"

Now, Gay Hendricks has taken a fresh look at the problem, and his research has generated an innovative solution. He has developed a simple program that gets excellent results very quickly. By focusing on physical flexibility, breathing, and relationship flow, even the most exhausted low-energy person can make a noticeable difference in his or her well-being in seven minutes a day.

In addition, he makes insightful recommendations for keeping our minds sharp with a program he calls Neuro-Gymnastics®. He also explores dietary principles for avoiding digestive energy-drains and for making food the enlivening fuel it should be.

As a doctor, I'm thrilled to have this book to hand my patients! The steps are medically sound and easily accomplished. We cannot ignore our bodies and expect to feel energetic. It's often the simplest things that go overlooked. We are meant to be moving, bending, and stretching regularly, and it's no surprise that our sedentary bodies don't feel energetically alive. We simply have to move and breathe consciously in order to get the most out of life, and Dr. Hendricks places this necessity at the very center of his program.

Likewise, we cannot ignore our diet and expect to feel alive. Simply put, we cannot put excessive amounts of heavily processed, chemical-laden, fat-and-sugar-rich food into our bodies and expect to feel good. Based on his research, Gay shows us that how we *feel* after we eat certain foods tells us how energy-producing (or energy-draining) those foods are. Being aware of this connection provides a new way for us to stay at our optimum weight.

I never paid attention to my own breathing or my patients' breathing until I discovered Gay Hendricks' work. Since then, I have used conscious breathing practices to reduce tension and stress build-up in my own body, and I've been able to help my patients reduce pain and anxiety using these same simple techniques. You will be amazed at how alert and energetic you'll feel if you take a moment now and then to practice the activities in this book.

Gay Hendricks, along with his wife and creative partner, Dr. Kathlyn Hendricks, is perhaps best known for his work in the area of relationship enhancement. Every day in my practice I see the cost of negative, dishonest relationships on health and well-being. Positive energy flow with people around us is essential to feeling fully alive, and Gay brilliantly shows how to achieve and maintain this flow in the simplest way possible.

The genius of *Achieving Vibrance* is in its ease and simplicity. As is so often true in life, tiny adjustments can make enormous differences. You won't have to make any large alterations in your lifestyle, and the few minutes you devote to this program will heighten your awareness and bring huge rewards.

Give yourself the gift of a few minutes a day to bring vibrance into your life. It's the way human beings are meant to feel, and now there's a simple program that makes it achievable.

Gay Hendricks changed my life, and he will change yours.

Achieving Vibrance

A PERSONAL MOTIVATION

In 1995, I took a good look at my life and didn't like what I saw. A friend of mine passed me at the airport as I was returning from a book tour and blurted out, "You're aging too fast!" At first I got defensively miffed at her comment, but then I looked in the mirror and saw she was right. (Nineteen cities in twenty-one days can do that to you!) I was beginning to look and feel old. I weighed 230 pounds, 50 more than my ideal weight. My low back and left knee and foot hurt most of the time. I was also feeling bored in my career and my marriage. I took an uncomfortable peek into the future and winced at what I saw: If I continued along the same path, I would "celebrate" my sixtieth birthday obese, virtually crippled, and creatively burned out. I would also be a relationship expert tired of his own marriage. It was a painful picture to contemplate.

THE QUESTION

So I decided to do something about it. Sitting in my garden one day, I hatched a radical question: What would it take for me to feel better *each day* than I felt the day before? What would I need to do, think, say, and feel to wake up lighter, clearer, more creatively vibrant—and more in love—than when I woke up the day before? With these questions in mind, I began to study carefully what I was doing that was causing me to rust out in my body, mind, and spirit.

First, like any good researcher, I dug into the literature on aging. I also visited numerous experts in the field and sorted through the truly vast array of products, nostrums, and supplements that populate the longevity marketplace. This experience was incredibly useful, but not for the reasons I first imagined. I was disturbed by the way the field was dominated by pharmaceutical companies and to a lesser extent by the vitamin industry. There is an old saying that I felt applied very well to the whole field: If the only tool you have is a hammer, everything looks like a nail.

Because of the vast profits to be made from drugs and vitamins, nearly everything being studied related in some way to the act of swallowing pills. I'm by no means an anti-pill zealot. For example, I take thyroid hormone every day because of a genetic disposition toward a sluggish thyroid gland. I also take Vitamin C and a multi-vitamin. However, if you walk through the exhibition hall at a longevity conference, I predict you will be overwhelmed by the thousands of different remedies being marketed. I also discovered a surprising irony in my research-travels on the longevity-circuit: Longevity experts often look older than they should for their age. There are some exceptions, of course, but I was often amazed by how stressed and prematurely old many of the experts looked. In one extreme example, one expert I thought was pushing seventy turned out to be fifty-two.

These observations led me to an even more radical set of questions:

- If funding the research were not an issue, what materials, tools, and techniques would be studied?
- If there were as much money to be made from non-pill solutions as from selling pills, what solutions would be offered?

I had many off-the-record talks with longevity experts on these matters. I concluded that just about everybody had some useful tidbit to offer, but nobody had anything definitive or magical. So I decided to start from scratch, and I'm very glad I did.

Throughout the development of the Vibrance program, we were guided by a very useful question: Is this the simplest possible way? This question led us to a profoundly different set of solutions. Much of the research on aging suffers from two problems: 1) It's too theoretical to be of much use to real people and their problems, and 2) it's heavily sponsored by pharmaceutical companies, thus slanting the "discoveries" toward pharmaceutical solutions.

For example, in a study of low moods, one group of people took an antidepressant, while a second group took a placebo pill. To control for the effects of being in an experiment (the so-called Hawthorn effect), the scientists taught a third group a simple technique borrowed from yoga. The technique was elegantly simple and entirely natural: When you notice your low mood, take three deep breaths, flex, and stretch.

The results were as unexpected as they were powerful: The "breathing/stretching" group improved their mood just as much as those taking the antidepressant! Only the sugar-pill group failed to improve. However, at the end of the article in the medical journal, the scientists called for more research into the antidepressant, recommending that a larger, more expensive study be conducted. Mysteriously, they did not call for further research into breathing or stretching. A cynic might suggest two reasons for this seeming oversight: 1) Pharmaceutical companies spend more money on research than yoga teachers, and 2) pharmaceutical companies are more interested in promoting pills than natural solutions that rely only on organic (and also free and easy) body processes.

The Vibrance program was developed with none of those kinds of biases. We were simply interested in learning what worked.

VIBRANCE:
A PROCESS AND A PROGRAM

As a process, vibrance is the art and science of increasing your clarity, ease, and vital energy each day. Vibrance is the main sensation you feel if you're *youthing* instead of aging. You're *youthing* if you feel more energetic, clear, and easeful today than you did yesterday. If not, you're aging. As a program, Vibrance is a few minutes of simple activities you do every day to produce energy, clarity, and harmony.

In the Vibrance program, you produce those results by conscious design, rather than allowing the default programming of unconscious aging to take over. On a moment-to-moment basis, you learn to make five mindset-shifts, which transform the experience of aging into a journey of vital expansion. These specific shifts directly counter the default programming that turns those years into a journey of contraction and creeping decay.

In the Vibrance program, you take responsibiity for how you feel each moment, and you take action with a series of flexes, breathing activities, and other bodymind processes. As your vital energy increases from within, your outer appearance changes dramatically. Within a few days, you'll feel the glow of vibrance happening inside you—within a few weeks, it becomes visible to your friends.

What we need to realize is that our vital energy can be turned on afresh at any age. The process of recovering our zest is part physical, part mental and emotional, part relational. More importantly, however, it is completely do-able.

Several paramount factors are at play:

- In our original youth, our spines could move through their full range of motion. With the Vibrance program, you regain that full range of motion in two minutes a day of a gentle innovative movement. We've seen chronic neck and back pain disappear after only a few minutes of learning the Vibrance-Flex.

- In our original youth, our breathing was free and deep and could nurture us with its calm energy. Then, we entered the world of critical people, air pollution, and emotional stress. By adulthood hardly anyone feels the energy and joy of healthy, free breathing. With the Vibrance program, you re-create your free breathing in two minutes of daily practice with a specific activity called the Vibrance-Breath. In a month or so, your breathing will almost certainly work better than the day you walked into elementary school.

- In our original youth, we were more likely to greet each moment with a creative, inventive mindset that allowed us to remain open and flexible in our thinking:
  - We wondered about the big questions, instead of accepting the answers of others.

Introduction

- We explored the new and unfamiliar, instead of shrinking back in fear.
- We felt our joys and sorrows deeply, yet could let them go and move on.
- We were in harmony with our natural rhythms—eating when hungry, resting when tired.

- In our original youth, we didn't hold as long to relationship regrets and resentments. We knew how to let go so we could re-awaken the flow of loving connection. We knew how to reach out for heartful connections, unless or until our natural urge to connect was thwarted by rejection.

By adulthood these natural processes of life often have come to feel alien instead of familiar. As a result, we often feel like strangers to ourselves. The Vibrance program gives you the power to re-create the same natural processes that many of us leave behind as we age. It gives you a new way to restore your birthright—a flow of natural energy you can feel every day.

CHAPTER ONE

Vibrance

What It Is and Why It's So Important

BEFORE I PUT ON MY AUTHOR'S HAT, let me speak first as the best customer. I use the ideas and techniques of *Achieving Vibrance* every day—I can't imagine my life without them. Here's why I'm such a passionate devotee.

At fifty I was stuck in a rut. I felt rusty, fat, and bored with my life, my work, and my marriage. Now, just a few years later, everything has changed. I've shed 50 pounds. I'm back in love with my wife and my life. My blood pressure is normal, my back pain has disappeared, and the creative wave I'm riding in my work is bigger than the one I surfed in my thirties and forties.

I feel better than I've ever felt in my life.

I owe this transformation to practicing the techniques in the Vibrance program, the exact same program you'll learn in this book.

THE VIBRANT PATH

As we set out together on the path to vibrance, I compliment you on your excellent taste and good common sense—you've chosen to embark on a unique adventure and a journey of limitless possibility. The vibrant way is important, even essential, and here's why: Every moment of every day, and every interaction with every person we meet, is flavored by our vibrance. When we feel our own natural vibrance, our contributions to others have greater depth, value, and meaning.

When we feel vibrant, we infuse each moment with the pure joy of being. When we are feeling the flow of vibrance inside us, we not only enjoy an enhanced sense of well-being in ourselves, we create an opening for others to expand into their own natural vibrance. In a very real way, giving the gift of vibrance to ourselves extends the gift to others at the same time.

Imagine a vibrant chef—glowing with high energy, good cheer, and clarity—emerging from the kitchen to place a gourmet meal before you. Now, imagine the same chef emerging from the same kitchen with the same dish—but this time the vibrance is missing. A weary scowl hangs on his pasty face as he slouches over to your table, slams down the dish, and lurks in the background to watch you eat it. Which meal do you think would taste better?

It's vibrance that makes life worth living.

The Journey to Vibrance

The journey to vibrance has a distinct advantage over other kinds of trips. If you go to a wondrous place such as the Grand Canyon, you have to wait until you get there to experience the big pay-off. With the wondrous journey to vibrance, you get to enjoy the big pay-off in every moment along the way. The techniques you'll discover in the Vibrance program produce a specific feeling in your body—the organic flow of vital energy—and you get to feel that flow a little bit more each time you practice the program. Can you spare seven minutes?

If you can, I can make you a life-changing prediction: Seven minutes of the Vibrance program will make you feel better all day and sleep better all night. No kidding.

I've made that prediction to hundreds of people as they began the program, and I'll make it to you. If you will invest a little time each day to do the program, you'll get a huge pay-off. Think of it as compound interest—a little bit of growth each day, but a substantial reward at the end of the year.

Let me go further with my prediction.

If you do seven minutes of the program today, you'll feel more vibrant than you did yesterday. If you do the Advanced program, you'll feel even more vibrant.

If you take seven minutes and do the program right now, you'll feel more vibrant than you felt seven minutes ago.

If you do it for a year, you'll feel better at the end of the year than you've ever felt in your life.

Although I've made these predictions to people well into their eighties, I've never had a single person come back and tell me my forecast didn't hold true. In other words . . . it works, it works reliably, and it works right away.

What Vibrance Feels Like

The feeling of vibrance *is a combination of vitality, harmony, and clarity.*

When you're feeling vibrant, you feel three sensations all at once:

- A pleasant flow of vital energy coursing through your body.
- A calm sense of integration, as if you're simultaneously at peace and all-of-a-piece.
- A spacious alertness of mind.

When we're feeling vibrant, we're present-centered and poised in keen readiness to engage openly with the world around us.

If there's a limit to how good you can feel using these techniques, we haven't discovered it yet. I feel better now in my mid-fifties than I've ever felt in my life, and most of the several hundred people we've studied say they do, too.

Not only does the program generate a unique feeling, it produces that result in an entirely new way. Vibrance uses all-natural, bodymind techniques instead of vitamins, medicines, or exercise. The techniques work immediately—you actually feel more vibrant within minutes. Although feeling good is great, Vibrance also turns heads: Our research found that other people start to notice your enhanced vibrance within a few days. Almost everyone who practices the program starts getting feedback that they're *looking* younger. This is excellent news for anyone, but particularly for the 70 million Americans who are over fifty and the 25 million more who will be turning fifty over the next few years.

HOW DID THE VIBRANCE PROGRAM COME ABOUT?

Working with 300 volunteers from ages 50 to 87 over a four-year period, my colleagues and I designed and refined a program by which feeling more vibrant by the day is not only possible, it's reliable and relatively easy. The title of the program was suggested by the participants themselves: After twenty-one days on the program, participants chose the following three adjectives (out of a page-long list) to describe the improvements they felt: *Vital, harmonious, clear.*

In the early days of the program, it took about 45 minutes a day to get these kind of results. As we refined the techniques, however, the efficiency of the program grew by leaps and bounds. Now, you can get major enhancements of your vibrance with a seven-minute basic program or a 15- to 20-minute advanced program. (It's important to note that the activities in the programs are so gentle and easy that we've had octogenarians do them every day for months with no injuries, stiffness, or pain afterwards. They're also simple to learn: Elementary school kids have taught them to each other effectively.)

A *Positive Focus*

I have never been comfortable with the combative stance of "anti-aging" or "fighting" free radicals. The combative approach may work in the wrestling ring or on the field of battle, but I don't think it's very useful in dealing with personal or social problems. Every time the government declares war on some problem (such as the "war" on poverty or the "war" on drugs), the problem seems to get worse. The same problem affects our inner world: Do we really want to "fight" our free radicals? If we really want to make free radicals disappear from our bodies, how about loving them to death?

Instead of going to war against our free radicals, let's put our energy into freeing our radical vibrance. Instead of fighting dis-ease, let's increase ease. Let's turn the whole endeavor in a positive direction. Let's put our energy into savoring and cultivating the actual feeling of glowing health. Let's shine a spotlight on the exact sensations that make us feel healthy—the flow of vital energy, harmony, and clarity—and then take positive actions to enhance that flow every day.

In my welcome pep-talk to people beginning the Vibrance program, I tell them, "Forget about increasing your life-span. Here, we focus on increasing our vibrance-span. Without vibrance, a long life is probably more of a curse than a blessing. Forget about 'anti-aging' or anti-anything-else. Here, we're *for* things— for harmony, for clarity, for increasing the flow of vibrance. If you feel more vibrant now than you did ten minutes ago, isn't that what's important? If you discover that the natural powers of your own bodymind can produce a felt-sensation of glowing health, isn't that what's important? You know in your heart, as I do, that having a long life is of no value whatsoever unless you feel the flow of vital energy."

THE MAJOR DISCOVERIES

In the course of working with over 300 men and women, ages 50 to 87, my colleagues and I made several important discoveries about what it takes to feel vibrant, especially as you get older. Our initial interviews focused on people over 50 and produced a treasure-trove of breakthrough insight. We found that maturing individuals do not fear death so much as they fear the diminished powers of decrepitude. As we looked into this problem further, we found that the fears were quite specific. People feared:

- Decreased physical energy.
- Mental fog.
- Disharmony, in the form of inner jangle and relationship turmoil.
- Decreased freedom and ease of movement, chiefly due to body pain.
- Relationship disharmony.

Achieving Vibrance

Once we had these variables identified, the "problem" of aging didn't seem quite so unwieldy. In fact, I felt a surge of positive energy—suddenly it seemed very do-able to find ways to make beneficial improvements in each of these areas.

My colleagues and I set forth to find new solutions to common problems. What we came up with were the following strategies to improve the areas most essential to living a vibrant life:

- *Physical Energy.* Experimenting with seventy techniques, we found a unique, gentle flexion movement that produces profound benefits in awakening a flow of physical energy while simultaneously reducing body pain. We found that it only needs to be done two minutes a day for results to be felt and seen.

- *Mental Clarity.* Researching thirty other techniques, we discovered a specific breathing practice that produces an immediate shift in mental clarity and emotional harmony. We found that between one and two minutes of the practice reliably produces the result. We also designed a program of quick and interesting mental activities, Neuro-Gymnastics. The activities enliven the mind and contribute to mental sharpness. Neuro-Gymnastics activities can be done any time of day and require no equipment or sophistication to perform.

• *Relationship Harmony.* We found that several specific actions restore relationship harmony and enhance the flow of relationship connections. We developed a simple way to teach these actions so that people—even those with no psychological knowledge or sophistication—could apply them to their daily lives.

• *Vibrant Nutrition.* We discovered a new way of eating that produces a feeling of vibrance, clarity, and stability. Although we did not set out to devise a weight-loss technique, we discovered that people who base their diet on "Vibrance-Foods" and eat according to "Vibrance-Timing" lose three to five pounds the first week they do so.

The Macarthur Foundation Study

In an unexpected way, my study of vibrance was inspired by the Macarthur Foundation Study. Like most people interested in the phenomenon of aging, I eagerly followed the Macarthur study of successful elders. It was a major research effort on a subject of compelling interest to every person on earth. The project consumed an enormous amount of money and the energy of many talented people. When the results were published, I felt two jarringly paradoxical emotions: excitement and disappointment. The overall finding was positive, provocative, and fit my own perceptions: Successful aging has almost *nothing* to do with genetics and almost *everything* to do with the psychological and physical choices you make every day. At the same time, however, the study was vague on the practicalities. In spite of all the tens of millions of dollars spent, the study told us very little about the microscopic level of how-to, what-to, and when-to. It was as if they had interviewed a thousand physically fit people coming out of a building but forgot to ask them if it was weight-lifting or ballet that kept them in shape. My disappointment was profound: How could a project of this magnitude have produced so much hope and so little useful information?

The Macarthur research tells us we should:

- Eat healthy, don't smoke, and avoid excess alcohol consumption.
- Do gentle exercise, because it works as well as its vigorous cousin.
- Have good relationships.
- Keep your mind alive by using it every day.
- Be extremely skeptical of the claims for "anti-aging" supplements, vitamins, and hormones.

Considering the millions of dollars and thousands of researcher-hours spent in gaining this information, the Macarthur study provided few of the juicy answers I'd been expecting. However, the Macarthur project motivated me, by its limitations, to go about my own study of conscious aging in a completely different way. I spent less than $100,000 on my project, relying instead on several dozen volunteer research-assistants and several hundred participants who gave their time in exchange for learning all of the techniques as we refined them. Metaphorically speaking, I chose a magnifying glass rather than a space telescope to study the subject.

Conclusion

Vibrance views the bodymind not as a machine but as a unified energy system. Our bodymind is a whole system with its own built-in resources for vibrant health, and those resources can be activated by techniques from inside the system. The results are created by improving energy flow in many dimensions, using the organic bodymind wisdom you already possess. Based on a new paradigm, *Vibrance* is unique—it opens your access to a hidden wellspring of well-being, giving you ownership of a natural resource most of us don't know we have.

Now, let's take a close look at just what that resource can give us.

CHAPTER TWO

How We Lose Vibrance, and How We Can Get It Back Again

≋≋≋

WHAT REALLY MATTERS each moment of our lives? Is it our work? Our relationships? Our health?

Certainly all of those are important, but my studies have shown me that it's really something much more fundamental. In a word, what matters is *vibrance*—the feeling of vital body-energy combined with a clear mind, emotional harmony, and an open heart. Lose your vibrance and you're old at 22. Feel your vibrance and you're young at 92.

Although vibrance feels incredibly good, there's nothing special about it. In fact, vibrance is our natural state, the way we're designed to feel. Vibrance says "Yes!" to life. When we're feeling vibrant, the day beckons us with possibilities: creative projects to be done, heart-connections to be made with people we care about. When we're vibrant we hum. When vibrance fades—when sludge has crept in—we say "No" to life or at best "Maybe later." We do the same old things and think the same old ways. We pull back from nurturing connection with others. We rattle in the places we used to hum.

Do you feel vibrant this moment?

How long has it been since you really hummed?

I asked myself those questions a few years ago and came up with two answers that scared me. The answer to the first question was "No." To the second, "It's been a while."

My vibrance had turned to sludge. I felt a rusty sluggishness instead of an inner glow. Instead of feeling clear, my mind often felt foggy and hopped around like a toad. Instead of emotional harmony, my heart often dragged. Sometimes a jangle of anxiety clanked with me everywhere I walked. My lower back, my knees, and my left heel also hurt, but those pains seemed trivial compared to the life-and-death feel of the sludge.

There's no question that sludge is costly. At Duke University, several hundred people over the age of 60 were studied for ten years, in order to find out what really contributes to health and disease as we age. Smoking cigarettes and being overweight were two main culprits, of course, but these two factors were not as important as something else: Moving your body! This huge study, costing millions of dollars and thousands of researcher-hours, revealed that physical inactivity is more likely to put you in the hospital than smoking or overeating. Physical inactivity turned out to be more lethal than we'd ever suspected: In the

Duke study, 50 percent of the physically inactive people died sooner than actuarily predicted.

Fortunately I woke up in time and de-sludged myself. I dug deep to find out what had happened to my hum. It took a lot of experimentation, first with myself and my colleagues, and then with several hundred others my age and older. Within a fairly short time, I turned off the sludge machine and recovered my hum. You can, too. All it takes is your commitment and the right tools.

Commitment is the important first step. You have to say, "Yes, I want to feel vibrant all the time, and I'll do what it takes to make it happen." You have to say it and mean it. That's the commitment I made, and that's the commitment I ask everyone to make who begins our Vibrance program.

I ask you to make it right now. If you'll make the commitment, the rest is easy. You're holding in your hands a powerfully effective toolkit that turns on a flow of vibrant vital-energy so fast it will amaze you.

Make the commitment and give yourself the gift of 10 to 20 minutes a day to do the program. It's never too late to begin. You may *think* it's too late, but that's your sludge doing your thinking for you. That's not the real you, the vibrant you who's waiting to emerge.

If a bed-ridden octogenarian with an oxygen-tube in her nose can benefit from the program, so can you. If after ten minutes of doing the program she can lift her head up off the pillow and say, "I feel the energy flowing," just imagine what you can do! If a 55-year-old marathon runner and a wheelchair-bound 75-year-old can both do the same program for a week and come back to tell me they feel vibrance humming in them, I'll bet you can, too.

WHAT HOLDS US BACK

There is abundant evidence that a lot of people don't know what really matters. That's a shame, and it's also shamefully expensive. At the heart-and-soul depths of ourselves, we cannot afford to be ignorant of what really matters. In the not-so-deep pockets of our taxpayer-selves, we can't afford it, either. The costs are simply too great.

Despair—giving up on ever humming with vitality again—is our main barrier. Once the sludge has taken over, it feeds on itself and excretes despair. The rigid thought patterns that accompany despair keep it stuck in place. Once sludge has taken over, we tend to become smug know-it-alls, and I can speak from experience as a recovering smug know-it-all of the first rank. See if you can top this for sheer arrogance: Thirty years ago I told a kindly friend that my life was going great. The "I" who said things were great was overweight, smoking heavily, and miserable in a troubled marriage. And yet I was telling the other fellow that things were just fine! Who was this "I" that thought things were going fine? That was my sludge talking, not the real me. From my sludge's perspective, I actually *was* doing just fine—the sludge was growing by the day! My friend was trying to save my life, and my sludge was telling him not to bother.

Fortunately I got a second chance, and you can, too.

For many years I've been studying what really matters as people get older. First, of course, I found a great deal to study in myself. Responsible doctors must be willing to take their own medicine, and responsible researchers must use their own bodies and minds as the initial field of discovery. I did so, and the experience made me feel younger and healthier than ever before. My team went on to study hundreds of people from 50 to 87 years of age, and we had many seemingly miraculous transformations along the way. I'd like to tell you exactly what we found. Then I'll show you how you can put the discoveries to work for you so that you'll wake up tomorrow feeling better, even if you feel great today.

THE ENERGY PRIORITY

Vital energy is the first priority. The first thing that really matters when you wake up each day is the feeling of vibrant energy flowing inside you. Lose it and you lose the zest for living. Our studies revealed something crucial: If you don't know how to turn on the flow of vital energy through natural methods, you'll try to remediate the lack by unnatural and costly means such as excess caffeine and sugar consumption, unnecessary purchases or trivial busy-ness. Without a felt-sense of vital energy moving in us, we slide toward despair. Despair is the bitter enemy of vibrance, especially in the years from midlife on.

What turns on the flow of vital energy? What turns it sludgy?

Here's what we know for sure, beginning with the two things that make you feel sludgy within minutes and even seconds if you don't pay attention to them:

- A specific way you move your spine turns on a feeling of flowing vital energy within two minutes. Our spines need to be flexed every day in all dimensions in order to stay lubricated and free. Human beings haven't been sedentary very long. If you think of all of evolution as a seven-story building, we humans occupy an amount of time equal to the coat of paint on the roof. And if you think of all *human* evolution as that same building, the amount of time humans have been sitting on furniture is even thinner than that coat of paint. We're born to move, to flex, to stoop to the ground and reach for the sky.

  The bottom line is this: If you don't move your spine through its full range of motion every day, you'll start feeling sludgy. A little bit of gentle movement is all it takes, and if you do a specific movement it can be done remarkably fast. I'll show you an elegantly simple movement you can do to turn on the flow of vibrance. You can even do it sitting at your work-desk, standing in a crowded elevator, or driving in your car. We've tested it out on thousands of people, and it works like magic. I'll also give you some advanced ways to do it if you have a little more time and want to feel really vibrant. They feel so good that our volunteers found they soon become a "positive addiction," to use the phrase coined by William Glasser, M.D. I predict you'll come to think of it as the most important two minutes you spend all day.

- You'll feel sludgy very quickly if the delicate flow of your breathing is hindered. Imagine how your car would run if someone tampered with the flow of air through your carburetor or stuck a potato in your exhaust pipe. Your breathing is designed to eliminate around two-thirds of the "exhaust fumes" from your body, compared to a third by all the other channels of elimination such as sweat and urination. Your breathing will do its job brilliantly well—if it's done correctly.

The bottom line is this: Vibrance depends a great deal on breathing. If you breathe correctly, you'll keep a proper balance between oxygen and CO_2 in your body. When those two are in harmony, you feel steady, calm, and energetic. When they are out of balance, you feel off-center. I'll show you a rapid way to reset the balance of your breathing when it gets thrown off-kilter by overwork and the tensions of everyday life.

THE CLARITY PRIORITY

Vibrance also depends greatly on how we use our minds. Our minds get troubled and smoggy when we operate them unwisely. For example, if we focus attention on things we can't control— whether people like us, what happened in the past, what will happen in the future—this mis-direction of focus generates rattle. The reason is simple: The mind is designed to solve problems; if you focus on something you can't change, you're giving it an unsolvable problem to solve. Faced with this dilemma, it jumps around until exhausted or spins out of control until you give up and shift your focus. When you shift to focusing on things you can control—what you can do for people, what you put in your mouth the next time you're hungry, what you can do today to make amends for past actions, what plans you can make today to make a better future—your mind settles down very nicely.

The grip of habitual thinking is another mental smog-producer. When we greet the new day with the same old mind, the results are pretty predictable. In actual fact, every moment we face is brand-new and calls for spontaneity of thinking. Our research discovered that there are five troublesome habit-patterns that cause most of the problems. I'll show you a simple way to break up those habits through specific conscious mind-shifts.

THE HARMONY PRIORITY

Relationships matter greatly in our daily lives. Failing to pay attention to several key relationship issues will make us feel so sludgy we won't want to get out of bed in the morning:

- Regrets—those things we feel bad about from the past and haven't yet cleared up with the significant person— eat away at our vibrance.

- Resentments also play a major role—the anger we cling to, the irritations we haven't expressed or released.

- A third relationship factor sounds easy but actually may be the most difficult—seeking out heartful connections. The modern world is arranged completely differently from the way it's been for hundreds of thousands of years. Even in the past hundred years, our society has turned upside down. When my grandmother was born in 1880, nineteen out of twenty people lived on farms. Now, nineteen out of twenty people live in cities and towns. That's a huge change in a short time, and we haven't caught up yet. We haven't yet learned how to reach out to other people in ways that give us the richness of identity that people felt not so long ago.

As an example, listen to the experience of Sidney, 67:

Before I started the program, I could probably be described as a lonely person. In the four years since my wife died, I had probably spent less than an hour all-told in any kind of intimate conversation with anybody. In the program, I realized that I was carrying a load of regrets and resentments that was keeping me from reaching out to certain family and friends. Once I started doing the ten-minute program, especially the minute where you consciously let go of regrets and resentments, I started being able to connect with people again. That seems like a miracle to me.

There is an art and a science to dealing with all these issues. I'll show you how to release regrets and resentments very efficiently—you can feel the immediate result in your body. I'll also show you a simple way to plan heartfelt connections with people you care about.

THE NUTRITION PRIORITY

How we eat can eat up our vital energy or enhance it abundantly. Specifically, what we eat produces either a vibrant feeling or a sludgy feeling, and that feeling will usually show up within a half-hour to 45 minutes after eating. I'll show you the simple art of eating for vibrancy. You won't ever have to spend another hour of your life feeling grumpy or out of sorts because of your nutrition or digestion. The first art of vibrant eating is choosing Vibrance-Foods. You'll see exactly how to do this in a later chapter, and I urge you to take the time. It's easy to do, and the instructions are given very specifically later on.

The second art of vibrant eating is learning to pay attention to a specific sensation in a specific spot in your body. Our research volunteers started calling it the V-Spot, in honor of its distant cousin, the G-Spot. Your V-Spot is about an inch below your zyphoid process, the soft indented place at the bottom of your sternum, and about an inch back toward your spine. Almost no one has any idea what I'm talking about when I first describe it to a group, but with a couple of minutes of training everyone I've ever worked with can feel it.

Why it's important is that the sensation in your V-Spot will tell you *exactly* when to stop eating. Your V-Spot will feel a pleasant sensation until you've had the perfect amount of food, then the pleasant sensation will disappear. If you stop eating right then, you feel vibrant. If you plow on through this body-signal and keep eating, you'll inevitably feel sludgy later.

Vibrance-Timing is the third art of vibrant eating. You are much more likely to stay vibrant throughout the day if you pay attention to when you eat. Specifically, we discovered that your vibrance is enhanced by eating a small amount of protein and complex-carbohydrate within a half-hour to 45 minutes after getting your feet on the ground in the morning. For example, I had a slice of apple and a couple of spoonfuls of yogurt at about 5:30 this morning after waking up at 5:10. You enhance your vibrance further if you then eat a larger portion of protein and carbohydrates within two hours after your "first-rising" snack. At

7:00, I had a bowl of high-fiber cereal and a little bit more yogurt. Our research into Vibrance-Timing also suggests that it's best to eat a complex-carbohydrate snack every couple of hours until your next meal. Simple carbohydrates—sugary or refined foods that are not accompanied by fiber—almost always decrease vibrance.

We've worked with people who say they've *never before* felt good after eating until they started eating Vibrance-Foods and paying attention to the V-Spot and Vibrance-Timing. They've told us that within a day of learning these two arts their bodies felt an awakening vibrance that was unique in their life experience.

A WHOLE SYSTEM IN FLOW

Since we are whole beings, not separate parts, everything I've mentioned is combined with everything else. For example, mental clarity and emotional harmony are twins that must be nurtured every day. By the same token, vital energy enhances both harmony and clarity. Energy, harmony, and clarity have an immediate effect on relationships. When people have handled the initial priorities of clear mind, inner harmony, and vital energy, they feel more of a desire to connect with others.

This brings us to . . .

THE AUTHENTIC SELF PRIORITY

The discovery of our authentic selves is an overarching priority in every phase of our lives. However, the need for it mounts in intensity as we enter our forties and becomes a life-or-death matter from 50 onward.

By the time we're 40 or so, most of us have developed a workable set of masks and acts. The very success of our masks is a strength, but it is also a handicap after 40. We have our Successful-Lawyer persona or our Dutiful-Parent act down pat. We had to master them to survive and prosper. However, after 40, and passionately after 50, life takes on a meaning beyond surviving and prospering. Notice that I'm not saying there's anything wrong with Successful-Lawyer or Dutiful-Parent or any other persona, mask, or act. That's the way life works: We're born with essence, we hide it under masks we need for surviving and prospering, then we uncover our essence again as we grow beyond the need to hide any of ourselves.

At a certain point in life, usually in our forties or fifties, we realize: *I have no further interest in concealing who I really am.* We decide: *I am only interested in discovering my true essence.* The good news is that the recovery of essence also brings youthful zest. There was a time you and I could play for hours with rapt focus and total immersion in the joy of the moment. Then we entered the world of school and work and attainment. This world required regimentation, discipline, and concealment. In fact, many of us discover to our dismay that the world of successful adulthood is built upon concealment. That rankles some of us, but we usually go along with the program.

When we get into our forties and fifties, we start getting feedback that even our most successful masks and acts are not bringing us fulfillment. When something isn't working, there is a human tendency to do it more. In other words, if our Successful-Lawyer act is not making us feel good inside any more, the human tendency is to go after a bigger case or a higher office in the bar association. Doing more of what isn't working has brought many people to my office. In my consulting-room over the past month, I saw two people who couldn't have been more different on the surface—but who had exactly the same classic post-50 issue:

- A celebrated entertainer—winner of awards, philanthropist, member of a powerful family—who is sick and tired of the world of fame. He calls it a "pretentious sham" and wonders if he will ever feel one moment of authentic love before his life is up. Before he caught on and came in for some coaching, he'd tried to override his lack of inner fulfillment by making four movies a year rather than doing one or two that he really liked.

  Fortunately he woke up in time. Now he's doing what he needed to do several years ago—embarking on the journey of discovering his authentic self. He thinks he may have waited too long to begin the journey, but I know it's never too late.

- A mother of four, who sweated her way up off welfare to a position of authority with a large government agency. Now that her children are grown, she's raising the question, "Who am I if I'm not serving others?" Even though she's loved and respected for her acts of service, she's wondering if there is anybody at home inside herself for *her.*

Suddenly one morning as she was waking up, she realized she was feeling a sense of despair in her body. She knew fear and she knew anger and she knew plenty of grief, but she was unfamiliar with the creeping sense of despair that people feel in their fifties if they do not set off on a quest for their authentic selves. Fortunately for her, she met this new sensation with a commitment to self-inquiry rather than a trip to the drugstore or the day-spa.

With that kind of commitment, she would get better even if she did nothing but stand next to a potted plant for an hour. With an hour of to-the-point coaching, however, she ignited a new glow of vital energy inside herself as she grasped her new life-purpose. Now she had a purpose that went beyond her pattern of serving others. Now she was committed to learning about her own needs and feelings and desires. This was unfamiliar territory to her, just as unfamiliar as her opposite number, a narcissist, might find a path of serving others.

THE ACTION PRIORITY

Purposeful actions characterize the vibrant person. If you know your purpose, your actions are guided by a through-line that makes you feel better about what you're doing. It doesn't matter if you are trekking through the Himalayas or sitting in a rocking chair, you need to know the purpose for doing the activity.

Purposeful action is an outgrowth of the quest for the authentic self. Purposeful action gives shape to our lives. Purposeful action requires that you know your purpose, both the larger purpose of your life and the more detailed purpose of your waking hours and minutes.

THE MOMENT-BY-MOMENT PRIORITY

Ultimately, vibrance will become who you *are*, but until then it's best to think of it as something you *do*. In fact, it is something you do every moment of every day by the way you handle specific life-situations. In working with successful people, we found that they make certain inner moves that contribute to their vitality. When faced with a choice between flexibility and sticking to a position for no good reason, the vibrant person chooses flexibility. Many people take arbitrary positions and stick to them. They do not practice flexibility of mind (or body), and it becomes a significant source of rust and decay. For example, I interviewed a man who'd eaten oatmeal for breakfast every day for thirty-four years. He had plenty of good reasons for it—many more reasons than oatmeal deserved, by my reckoning (and his wife's). His long oatmeal-streak was just one of many positions he stuck to. His wife said he was the most stubborn individual she had ever met. Now in his fifties, his rigidity was causing a lot of problems, ranging from back pain to relationship strains. He defended all of his positions vigorously—it was hard getting him to see that the very act of defending his positions *was* the problem. Some time early in his life, he'd survived by stubborn adherence to position, and he still thought it was the required way to do things, even in the face of abundant feedback to the contrary.

Another example: A man visiting my house observed me grinding coffee beans to make coffee. He sniffed the aroma and said it smelled delicious. He said he'd never seen anybody grinding his own beans before, adding that he always drank instant coffee for breakfast. He was a prominent fellow from an old-money family, so I knew it wasn't a financial issue that kept him from enjoying real coffee. I asked him if he'd like to try a cup of my brew, and he shook his head somewhat sadly and said "No." Noticing the "sad" body language, I asked him why he turned down the coffee. He said it was because he was afraid he might enjoy it—then he would feel bad about drinking what he "had to" drink for breakfast every day.

This point of view was upside-down from the way I live my life—I'm always on the lookout for little ways to improve the quality of my life. I was so curious about his position that I couldn't help pressing him further. I asked him: Why not try the new experience? If you enjoy it, let it inspire you to grind your own beans at home. Again, he shook his head sadly. He explained that by the time you get to be a certain age (he was about 55), you've got to stick with your habits. Plus, he said, his wife was used to making instant coffee, and it might upset her to "have to" change. If he asked her to change after thirty years, it would imply there had been something wrong with the way she'd been doing it.

Wow! Good thing Columbus didn't think like that—the ship would have cruised around the bay a couple of times, then headed back to the dock.

There are plenty of times in life when sticking to your position is a great thing—to stand up for a principle, to defend your home turf or loved ones, to push an important project through to completion. However, most of the positions that people take do not serve such grand and glorious purposes. They are more likely to be of the instant-coffee-and-oatmeal variety.

I said to my oatmeal-eater, "Would you rather your tombstone say 'He ate oatmeal every day for thirty-four years' or 'He had the courage to try new adventures'?" He got the point.

LIVING IN EXPANSION OR DYING IN CONTRACTION

If you feel an emotion emanating from your chest—perhaps sadness or longing—do you pause to give it your full attention or do you try to make it go away? It's an important question because the act of turning toward, rather than away from, emotionally charged experience is one of the defining characteristics of vibrant people. Specifically, they turn their consciousness *toward* their emotions and the situations that trigger those emotions. When fear grips their belly, they inquire into it by directing their focus toward the sensations in their gut. When a painful situation develops with a friend or relative, they reach for the phone to communicate about it rather than hoping it will go away. To use a car-metaphor, the vibrant person does not respond to a knock in the engine by turning up the radio to drown out the noise. The vibrant person listens to it carefully to find out what needs to be done.

SELF-FUL, NOT SELFISH

Vibrant people are *self-ful* but not *self-ish*. A participant in one of our research projects came up with the term "benign selfishness." By this she meant the crucial skill of learning to ask questions like, "Is this what *I* really want to be doing right now?" and "Is this really what *I* want for dinner tonight?" Our research team came to call this skill *essencing*, the act of discovering our true selves in each moment. We called it this because it gets to the heart of something that keeps us youthing as we age: the art of nurturing our essence—who we truly are—rather than continuing to conceal our true selves behind our masks or personas. There is no question that we need masks in order to move through life. The question is this: Do we really need to keep those masks on all the time? Vibrant people learn to remove those masks and initiate an ongoing search for the authentic self.

THE ART OF LISTENING

As we will explore in detail in our chapter on the Vibrance Mindset, listening plays a major role in the lives of vibrant people. Vibrant people tend to be generous listeners. They draw the other person out through the quality of their listening. By contrast, non-vibrant people tend to engage in Mousetrapping, which is the conversational equivalent of a karate chop. It drops the conversation to its knees. If you are practicing what our research team calls "generous listening," you draw out the speaker through one beat after another. In other words, you demonstrate genuine interest. If the speaker says, "I'm having a great day," the generous listener asks, "Wonderful—what makes it so?" The Mousetrapper would respond to that same utterance with, "I sure wish I was."

INNOVATING INSTEAD
OF ROUTINIZING

Our research discovered that vibrant people go to great lengths to vary their routine. We uncovered many creative examples of innovating instead of routinizing. While some of them may sound trivial or ridiculous, they result in keeping people flexible and sharp:

- Putting on clothing a different way each day (i.e., left pants leg on first one day, right pants leg on first the next day).

- Going to the same place by a new route.

- Calling someone who usually calls you.

- Leaving the television off all day . . . consciously not watching the news or a show you habitually watch.

- Brushing your teeth with the "wrong" hand (this seemingly silly activity—which one of our subjects called 'brushin' roulette'—turned out to be one of the favorite methods for reliably triggering a brightening of mental clarity). You'll learn more about these in our chapter on Neuro-Gymnastics.

One powerful question set my quest for vibrance into motion: What are the essential things we must do if we want to wake up tomorrow feeling more vibrant than when we woke up today? This question means even more to me today than it did five years ago. Even though I feel immeasurably more vibrant than I did back then, I keep asking that question every day *because I keep feeling more vibrant every day I ask it.* I urge you to make it the organizing principle of your daily life.

The answers you'll find in this book may surprise you. All I ask is that you try them out. Solid scientific evidence supports every element of the program, but that's not what really matters. What matters to you is that you feel better tomorrow than you did today—even if you feel fine today. If you keep doing that, day after day, you'll find as we did that the magic works: There's no upper limit on how good you can feel and how creative you can be.

VIBRANCE IN ACTION: A CASE STUDY

For a living example of how vibrance can work and keep on working, come with me on a visit to one of the most vital people in my study, Laura Huxley, who also is our senior participant in terms of chronological age.

My wife, Kathlyn, and I visited Laura at her lovely cottage in the Hollywood hills. At 87 on the day we visited, Laura is the very embodiment of vibrance. A successful author and speaker in her own right, Laura is also the widow of novelist Aldous Huxley.

Laura radiates a key principle of vibrance: We "youth" ourselves by flexing our mind, body, and spirit every day. As we talked, Laura's yoga teacher sat nearby. Laura was planning to do an hour of yoga as soon as we left. Laura's first priority every day is to extend her body's flexibility by stretching, yoga, and other practices. As I sat talking to Laura, I noticed a trumpet sitting on a nearby table. I knew Laura played violin in her early days, but

I'd never heard of her blowing a trumpet. I asked her about it, and my heart leapt when I heard her answer. She said she'd just bought it but hadn't yet learned to make a sound with it. I was impressed: The trumpet is notoriously difficult to play, and she was taking it up for the first time at 87! Here is another key principle of vibrance in action: Learning something new every day re-creates the flow of youthful energy.

I played trumpet when I was a kid, so I picked Laura's new instrument up and blew a few phrases on it. "That's my goal," she said in her lovely Italian accent, "Just to make one sound that is beautiful." I helped her get a few sounds out, and in doing so I noticed some problems with the way she was breathing while trying to play. I showed her how to make the sound stronger by breathing from her diaphragm rather than up high in her chest. This made an immediate difference in the quality of the sound but also in her overall feeling of well-being. (This is not surprising—in many research studies of aging, the key variable that's measured is vital capacity of breathing.)

As I mentioned in the last chapter, listening plays a key role in vibrance, and Laura is a consummate practicioner of the art. She, like many vibrant people, has a way of listening deeply to people, so that the speaker has permission to speak freely and deeply.

Some people listen so that it puts the brakes on what the other person is saying. Here's an example, exaggerated for effect, but not too different from many I've heard as a therapist over the decades:

WIFE: Honey, while you were at work today I had a life-changing enlightenment experience in which I accessed my full creative potential and decided to move to Oregon to join a poetry commune.

HUSBAND: What's for dinner?

The husband slammed the brakes on the conversation by switching abruptly to his own needs and feelings. Think of what a different marriage this would be if he'd said, "It sounds like a powerful experience. Tell me more."

Vibrant people tend to listen with genuine curiosity. Here's an example from our visit with Laura Huxley.

ME: Have you ever tried playing the shakuhachi?

LAURA: No, I haven't. What is it?

ME: It's the bamboo flute played in Zen monasteries in Japan. Beautiful sound but pretty hard to play. You really have to use your diaphragm.

LAURA: You think it would help my breathing?

ME: It sure helped mine. You really can't get a decent sound out of it unless you're doing a deep, slow diaphragmatic breath. It's good training.

LAURA: I wonder where I would get one around here.

ME: I'm going to find one and get it to you.

At no point did she interrupt the flow to ask "What's for dinner?" I later rewarded her curiosity by gifting her with one of my flutes. (A magical aside: I talked about my visit with Laura to musician Kenny Loggins, my friend and Santa Barbara neighbor. He later surprised me with a gift from his collection, a wonderful handmade shakuhachi to replace the one I'd given Laura.)

Whenever I think of the worst kind of listening, I recall one of my fellow-professors at the University of Colorado, where I taught for twenty-one years. His consummate narcissism was already legendary by the time I arrived on campus, and he maintained a nearly flawless record as a poor listener the entire time I knew him. At first I was surprised, because he was the author of various books on therapy and communication skills. Here are a couple of interchanges.

ME (BACK FROM SPRING BREAK AND FEELING EXUBERANT): We had a fantastic time in Aspen.
HIM: It rained the whole time in Cancun. A total bummer.

On another occasion, we were both getting our mail out of the faculty boxes:

ME: Is this what I think it is? (I excitedly rip open a package containing my newly published book. I pull the book out and study the cover. He glances and turns away.)
HIM: I wish I had time to write these days.

You can probably see why people who listen like that tend to rust as they age, as well as suffer for lack of friends.

Achieving Vibrance

By contrast, Laura demonstrates interest in everything around her. In addition, she actively cultivates a flow of relationship connections. She operates a foundation from her cottage, bringing many young people by to visit, and she has a rich network of friends she stays in contact with. Recent visitors had been Ram Dass, recovering from a stroke at the time, and Artie Shaw, former clarinet superstar of the swing era.

As we left, her thirty-four-year-old yoga teacher said, "Laura, I want to be like you when I'm 87." My wife, Kathlyn (over three decades younger than Laura), said, "I want to be like her *now!*"

CHAPTER THREE

The Vibrance-Mindset

Specific Attitudinal Shifts That

Increase Your Vibrance

≈≈≈

I'VE BEEN RICHLY BLESSED to know several hundred people who were enjoying both maturity *and* vibrance. I didn't find them by accident—I went looking for them, inspired by motivations I'll describe shortly. What I discovered through talking with them opened up a whole new world of possibilities.

I began my study of people over 50 the same year I turned 50. The years since then have been in every way the most rewarding of my career as well as my life as a whole. Whoever said "Life begins at 50" got it right, indeed.

In my experience, vibrant maturity is life at its best. What could be better than feeling great while enjoying the wisdom earned through life experience? Of course, I know many people don't feel this way. In my therapy practice, I've counseled hundreds of people at midlife who were dreading or lamenting the years in the second half of life. Before I turned 50 myself, I listened to them, empathized with them, and did my best to help them find solutions to the problems with which they were struggling. When I turned 50, though, I became much more than a sympathetic listener—I became highly motivated to find ways to make my own life more vibrant as I matured.

Flashback . . . to a few days after my fiftieth birthday: I have a vivid memory of opening my mailbox and finding an unexpected gift, my very own copy of *Modern Maturity*. For those who may not know, this fine magazine is published by the American Association of Retired Persons. Before that day, my only association with *Modern Maturity* was in my dentist's waiting room. There was always a plentiful supply of them scattered around, but in spite of their abundance I'd picked them up about as often as I remembered to floss. I associated the magazine with "old folks" because it was "them" I usually saw reading it in the waiting room. Suddenly, standing by my mailbox that day, the realization hit me: I'd become one of "them."

I grimaced and started to toss the magazine in the trash. Then I caught myself in mid-toss, wondering why I had grimaced at an innocent magazine—one I hadn't even opened. I remember thinking, "Maybe there's a message here somewhere."

I paused right there in front of my mailbox and decided to confront whatever I'd been avoiding. I forced myself to open the magazine and scan the table of contents. Practically every title jumped out at me as something I was concerned with. I realized as I flipped through the pages that the magazine was a metaphor for issues of aging I did not want to address.

The next few days went by in a whirl of excitement as well as a stir of anxiety. I saw that I'd been avoiding thinking about turning 50 because I dreaded becoming what some members of my family had turned into as they aged. When I explored my fear more deeply, I realized more specifically what I was afraid of. Except for my grandparents and one aunt, every member of the generation ahead of me had become more difficult to be around in their years after 50. It wasn't their physical infirmities that caused the difficulty—in fact, often the only way I could connect with them was around a physical ailment such as taking them to the doctor or helping them stand or sit.

The real problem was in the change in their mindset and personalities. With several family members, their tobacco and alcohol addictions got worse as they grew older. They were harder to talk to and more volatile in mood. In addition, of course, they also suffered more sickness that smoking and drinking causes. I saw another family member get more stubbornly rigid, wrapping herself more tightly inside the bondage of her prejudices, judgments, and opinions. The stubbornness had always been there, but earlier it had been in a milder form that she and other people joked about. Between 50 and 70, though, it became no laughing matter. Eventually, hardly anybody in the family could stand to be around her for fear of triggering one of her rants about race, youth, or the decline of civilization, as especially exemplified by other members of the family.

I did not want to go down that path. I decided then and there to find a new path to maturity, one that made every step of the way something different and better than what I'd seen around me. That decision led me to seek out several hundred people over 50 who were having a great time. I spent the next four years talking to vibrant post-50 folks with the big question in mind: How do they do it? I wanted to find out what they were thinking and doing to make their post-50 experience a journey of vibrance rather than a slouch into bitterness and decrepitude.

What these vibrant midlifers taught me changed my life. My big learning was this: Vibrant aging is not about genetics, IQ, education, or even health. It's not about luck, either: It's about the choices we make every day. Actually, it's about the choices we make *every moment.* I discovered that we can cultivate a vibrance-mindset if we make vibrant choices over time. This vibrance-mindset serves us admirably. As we move through the world, we remain poised in an always-ready stance of willingness to move into greater vibrance. Over time this mindset grows . . . and shows.

THE ELEMENTS

I'd like to share several key elements of the vibrance-mindset with you. There are probably more elements waiting to be discovered, but these five came prominently to light as I worked with several hundred vibrant people over the last few years. As I describe these elements, I'd like you to approach them with your bodymind—in other words, think physically as well as metaphorically.

For example, I call the first element "Flexing," and I contrast it with its non-vibrant opposite, Sticking-to-Position. This element has physical as well as metaphorical implications. First, think physically—picture yourself sitting in a chair watching TV for an hour without changing your position. When you finally stand up, you notice that you feel stiff and sluggish. Instead of flexing your body now and then to keep it limber, you stayed in one position for the whole hour. The failure to flex yourself had a specific result—you felt stiff and sluggish later.

The element also has a metaphorical aspect. Let's say I cling to some position in my mind, such as the attitude espoused by my beloved (and monumentally crusty) grandfather, "Washing dishes is women's work." To my knowledge, he never touched a wet dish in his ninety-three years. This attitude somehow works its way into me, causing me to resent doing dishes earlier in my life. However, I soon found that the women of my era had less tolerance for this position than my grandmother apparently had. If I hadn't demonstrated the flexibility necessary to let go of this position, my rigidity might have brought costly consequences upon my head.

The First Element: Flexing

This first element is a key to the other four, so we will explore it in careful detail. If you understand it and its powerful implications, you enjoy a genuine advantage on your journey to vibrance.

Begin by understanding this: There's a time for sticking to our positions, and there's a time for letting go of them. Vibrant maturity depends on knowing when to hold to a position and when to get flexible and try something new.

I consider that a position is worth sticking to under the following conditions:

- It serves your well-being.
- It does not deprive you of genuine growth opportunities.
- It facilitates relationship harmony among you and the people you love.
- It rests on a foundation of values and choices you've freely embraced.

Most of us have principles and beliefs that meet these criteria. These are the positions worth sticking to. For example, I developed a position about alcohol when I was in college. The first couple of times I drank beer with my buddies, I learned, from listening to my body, that I felt fine with half a bottle of beer in me. If I tried to finish a whole bottle, though, I felt off-center, sluggish, slightly irritated. My conclusion: Alcohol is a poison to my body in all but small doses. I noticed the same effect after one glass of wine. One glass felt fine—two felt like poison. In the decades since then, I've probably been asked several hundred times, "Aren't you going to finish that beer?" I shake my head and reply, "Nope, I'm a half-a-beer guy."

My half-bottle rule meets all the criteria for a principle

worth sticking to. It definitely serves my well-being. It's based on my own experience, and I chose it freely. There would be little or no growth opportunity in letting go of this position. (I suppose we could stretch the point and say I've missed out on experiences like being drunk or having a hangover. However, beyond increasing my empathy for drunks and hangover-sufferers, I'm not sure there would be any genuine growth for me in either of those experiences.)

Most people also have religious and moral positions that they consider worth sticking to. If you take comfort from believing that a heaven or a next incarnation awaits you after death, why not hang onto that belief? Even though beliefs like that are not based on experience, it's probably not costing you substantial growth opportunities to cling to it. The exception would be if you were using the concept of heaven or reincarnation to avoid facing some aspect of death. Also, some people cling to religious beliefs in ways that distance them from loved ones, but that has more to do with the individual's personality than the belief itself.

However, many of us also carry weighty baggage in the form of principles, beliefs, and rules that limit our growth opportunities and keep us from feeling vibrant. We often cling to these principles and beliefs out of fear. What's worse is that many of these limiting positions are not even based on our own experience.

One of the first things I learned from my study of vibrant post-50 folks is that they are nimble at letting go of unnecessary positions. I invite you, for the sake of your vibrance, to inquire boldly into the positions you hold. Let go of the ones that no longer serve you. Flex yourself into new positions that expand your growth opportunities in every moment.

How to Spot Your Limiting Positions

There are several ways to spot your limiting positions.

First and most important, listen carefully to the thoughts in your mind and the language you use. Take special note when you think or say:

> I can't . . .
> I don't . . .
> I'm too old to . . .
> I'm just . . .

In a few minutes of going through my session notes, I quickly found the following examples. They are so common that I probably could find hundreds more without exhausting the supply.

> I can't dance.
> I don't fly.
> I'm too old to do stuff like that (accompany his wife to a salsa lesson).
> I'm just not an exercise-person.
> I can't for the life of me learn a foreign language.
> I don't have an ear for opera.

I'm over 50 now, way too old to enjoy something like
that (accompany her husband on a trek to the
Himalayas).

I'm just the kind of person who gets sick a lot, I guess.

I'm just old-fashioned (using this as a reason she
wouldn't do a guided-imagery exercise with her husband in my office).

Notice the large number of "can'ts" and "don'ts" in those
examples. If you pay careful attention to your thoughts and
words, you'll probably be amazed, as I was, to discover how
many self-limiting shackles we apply to ourselves. Listening to
your own language will give you clear information about where
you're holding unnecessary positions. This endeavor can be
more challenging than it sounds. Often, the way we speak is so
habitual that it becomes virtually impossible to hear where we
are limiting ourselves. Fortunately, most of us have friends and
family around, and they provide us with another simple way to
find out where we're clinging unnecessarily to limiting positions.

The second important way to discover your limiting positions is this: Think of other people as mirrors. Our friends and
family members serve as mirrors to the aspects of ourselves we
can't see by self-observation. You may have noticed that friends
and family members tend to point out our limitations with
relentless regularity. It's easy to slough off this feedback by
blaming them for being critical. Indeed they often are, but it's
also important to acknowledge that we usually have a filter over

our ears that hears feedback as critical when it's really not. Also, even the most critical feedback has a grain of useful truth buried somewhere in its irritating midst.

This leads me to an important discovery I made about myself. The quickest and totally foolproof way to find out if I am clinging unnecessarily to a position is to notice if I get defensive about it. Take one of the examples I've given above: Suppose you come up to me and say, "Gay, I heard you say you can't dance. Don't you really mean that you're afraid to dance because you don't like to look silly? You *can* dance—you just don't want to."

My reaction would tell you immediately whether this was a position I was holding onto unnecessarily. If I responded in an undefended way, I might say something like this: "You know, you're absolutely right. Thinking I can't dance is just a thought— I could probably even enjoy dancing if I were willing to let go of that thought."

If I got defensive, I might say, "Nope, can't dance. Tried it in junior high school and fell flat on my face. Don't know why I can't dance—guess it's genetic."

My defensive reaction would be a clear sign that this position was an unnecessary, fear-based clench that was blocking growth opportunities. Sometimes the best thing to do is to move through the fear and do the thing we're afraid of. I've done that many times—from getting married to scuba diving—and I've never regretted it. However, I'm not saying we should always give up the clench and do the thing we're afraid of. Sometimes there are complicated reasons for continuing to hold an unnecessary position. What's important, though, is to know what those reasons are, so that if you continue to hold the position, you'll at least know why.

Let me give you an up-close example, involving two incredibly brilliant, self-sufficient women I knew well: my mother, Norma Hendricks, and my aunt, Audrey Williamson. My mother was a journalist and newspaper columnist, and my aunt was the administrator and speech writer for a senator for thirty years. They both succeeded in the (largely man's) world of twentieth-century America, and I feel very lucky to have been born into the same family as two such remarkable people. (By the way, both of them loved it when I have told stories about them in my books or on talk shows, so I'm sure they'd be delighted that I'm sharing this one.)

In 1979 I invited my mother, then 68 and in good health, to accompany me on a trip to England that I needed to make in about five months. I'd heard her say many times how much she wanted to visit the British Isles. The trip seemed like a perfect opportunity to spend some alone-time with her, something I hadn't done much as a grown-up. I sent a note, inviting her on the trip and giving her the dates. I felt so excited by the possibility that I don't think I considered for a moment that she might not want to go.

A week or two went by without a response. Mom was a great correspondent, and not to reply was so unlike her that I knew something was up. I called down to Florida to find out what was going on, and although she updated me on the weather and the medical status of her and her friends, she didn't bring up the subject of my invitation. Finally I said, "Mom, you haven't told me whether you can go to England with me." She grew flustered and said, "I can't do a thing like that."

Hearing my indomitable mother say "I can't" was so unfamiliar that it threw me for a loop. After all, this was a woman who had guest-piloted the Goodyear blimp, interviewed Elvis Presley, chatted up JFK, and with dead-eye precision shot a rattlesnake that had invaded our backyard. I asked her to explore her "I can't" with me. She said that her older sister, my aunt Audrey who lived next door, liked her coffee a certain way. Mom said she had started going to Audrey's house to make morning coffee and that Audrey wouldn't like it if she had to go back to making her own coffee for a week. My brain went on "tilt" at hearing this, and I recall staring at the phone in utter disbelief. My aunt was a renowned gastronome. She made the best cup of coffee I'd ever tasted. I could feel the "son" part of me want to argue with my mother by telling her how ridiculous her position was. Fortunately, by then I was also an experienced therapist, and this part of me won out over my argumentative "son."

I shifted from my head to my heart, knowing suddenly that our conversation had nothing to do with coffee. Her position had something to do with the bond between her and my aunt, and it was my job to understand it and resonate with it rather than talk her out of it.

As we talked, the emotional underpinnings of the position emerged. My aunt had always been the "big sister" against whom my mother had competed since the day she was born. The competition served them well, inspiring them to outdo each other in their achievements. But now, in retirement, they had finally resolved this issue. They were best friends now, on equal footing, and my mother simply didn't want to leave her best friend behind, even for a week. Audrey had done all the traveling she wanted to do, and she had made this position so clear for so long that it had not even occurred to me to invite her to go along with us.

Finally, after much discussion, I felt I understood the situation well enough to call the question: "It sounds like you want to decline my invitation." She said she did, and we left it at that.

Here's my point: Both of us were better off, in my opinion, after having explored the deeper foundations of the position. I could have swept her defensive move under the rug by not asking why she hadn't responded to my invitation. If I'd done that, though, there would have been a big lump under the rug of all our future conversations. We would both have known we were avoiding the issue. Also, had we not explored beneath the "coffee position," we would not have connected on the deeper emotional level that ultimately strengthened the bond between us.

If we are courageous enough to dive beneath the surface of our positions and our defenses, we open to new worlds of possibility. As in my mother's case, we may explore a position only to choose consciously to remain within its limitations. Or . . . we may go in a bolder direction: We may decide to slip free of the position's grip and soar into the unknown.

What if Mom had decided she wanted to go? What if she had simply told the truth to Audrey, "I want to go to England, *and* I don't want to leave you behind."

We'll never know what might have happened, but here are a few possible scenarios, based on many other similar situations I've encountered in my therapy office.

Audrey might have said, "Wow, that sounds like fun! I think I'll let go of my 'I've-seen-it-all' position and come with you!"

Or she might have said: "Go! I'll take a few days and go visit the Botanical Gardens, which I know you don't want to do."

Or she might have said: "I'm touched. Let's take a moment and acknowledge how close we've gotten and how grateful we both feel. Then you can go or not go, but we will know we've celebrated what's important."

Those are the kinds of options that open up when we start flexing out of our locked-and-defended positions. I came upon a radical example of flexing on the very trip in question. I spent a couple of days in Paris after my business in England was over. I was resting on a park bench in the Tuileries, sipping a cup of espresso, when a vibrant woman of my mother's age sat down beside me. We started chatting, and during the next half-hour my jaw dropped more than once. She told me she had just walked all the way from Portugal, a trek that had taken six weeks. That got my attention, but then she went on to tell me that she had started walking around the world when she retired two years before. First, she'd walked from Arizona to California, then decided she wanted to go the other direction! So, she walked back all the way to the east coast, taking the better part of a year to make the trek.

She said she'd asked her husband to come, but he'd declined on the grounds that he would miss his favorite TV shows. "I call him once a week," she assured me, "and he seems to be getting along fine without me." He'd flown out to visit her on a couple of occasions, then returned home to his version of the good life.

I offered to buy her a drink so I could hear more of her story, but she declined, saying she was getting itchy to get her sneakers (her sixth pair, by the way) into the Alps. I watched her stride briskly across the Tuileries into the next chapter of her vibrant life.

We all can benefit from asking ourselves questions like:

> What positions am I holding onto unnecessarily?
> How am I limiting my growth opportunities through clinging to positions?
> What could I become if I were willing to flex myself fully in every moment?
> What opportunities would come my way if I were fully flexible?

My wife, Kathlyn, and I came across a superb example of flexing when we were teaching a workshop at a California massage school and healing retreat center. I discovered to my surprise that one of the owners of the center, a man in his fifties, had been a powerhouse trust lawyer in Chicago. I asked him how such a radical transition had come to pass. It seemed a long way from the windy canyons of downtown Chicago to the sunny hills of Sonoma. He told me that it all started when he noticed how many of his clients died soon after retiring. One day he looked in the mirror and realized that the only reason he was still lawyering in Chicago was so he could someday retire to California. He felt an uncomfortable shudder pass through him: Was I going to be one of those who worked to 65, doing something I didn't want to do, then died the day after? He decided not to wait, and as soon as he made the decision the practical means seemed to open magically before him.

Standing in front of me was a happy man, wearing a pair of shorts, sandals, and a T-shirt. He was obviously Flexing instead of Sticking-to-Position. "Ever miss it?" I asked, already knowing the answer. He grinned and shook his head, off to his yoga class.

The Second Element: Heliotroping Instead of Contracting

You've probably seen heliotropes, a variety of flower that turns toward the sun. When the heat and light touches them, they open up to receiving the energy rather than shrink away from it. In conducting my conversations with vibrant people over 50, I noticed that they demonstrated a remarkable ability to turn toward—rather than shrink away from—things that were trying to get their attention. My colleagues and I began to call this ability *heliotroping* and contrasted it with its opposite, *contracting*. I regard it as one of the hallmarks of a vibrant mindset.

The sun is powerful energy. It's so far away that we can

hardly conceive of the distance, yet it can warm us, heal us, or burn us, depending on how we relate to it. Think of the sun as a metaphor for the kinds of powerful energies that occur in our lives day in and day out. For example, pain is a strong energy. I have some of that pain-energy in my feet as I write, reminding me of last night's dance-party with my wife and some of our colleagues. A geographical move, a sudden illness or the death of a loved one—all of these are powerful blasts of energy. All of them send shock-waves of anger, grief, and fear through us. Life is full of such waves of energy, and the intensity increases after 50.

The energy itself is certainly important: the pain, the grief, the move, or whatever. More important than the energy itself, though, is how we relate to the energy. How we relate to pain or grief or other strong energies tells us who we really are as human beings. Do we turn toward the energy to embrace it? Or do we shrink away from it in contraction? It's a choice presented to us in many moments of the day, in many experiences large and small.

Picture me and a dozen others lying on our backs on exercise mats, at the fitness class I attend. We are three-fourths of the way to a hundred stomach-crunches. All of us have put ourselves in this position voluntarily. Indeed, we've even paid for the privilege of being tortured in this particular manner. We are all participating in the same strong energy, yet each of us relates to it differently.

On either side of me I hear two very different reactions. On my right is a guy I think of as the Whiner. He likes to make sarcastic remarks when in pain. This time he gasps to our trainer, "Do you *haaaave* to go so fast?" Last class he said something similar, "Do you *haaaave* to sound like you're having so much fun making us hurt?" Some people in the class politely chuckle at his comments, but I notice that none of us ever invites him to join us when we hit the juice bar after class.

On my left is the Groaner. He likes us to hear how hard he's working, so he makes loud suffering sounds as he gets near the end. Me, I'm the Stoic. I take pride in being able to endure massive amounts of pain without a peep.

Which is better? I could make an eloquent case for the virtues of the Stoic approach. I could even quote long passages by heart from Epictetus and Marcus Aurelius, two of my favorite Stoics. But you know what? I bet my two mat-mates could make an equally strong case for their ways of relating to the strong energy. The Whiner could probably lecture us for hours about whining as a spiritual path. So could the Groaner. Nobody's way is right—they've all got pluses and minuses.

What I'm saying is: It's how we relate to the energy—in this case the increasing muscle-burn in our bellies—that defines our personalities. The way we go toward the energy—or turn away from it—tells us who we are at the core.

The great writer Hermann Hesse put it very well:

> Suffering only hurts because you fear it. Suffering only hurts because you complain about it. It pursues you only because you flee from it. . . . Do not resist it, do not flee

from it. Taste how sweet it is in its essence, give yourself to it, do not meet it with aversion. It is only your aversion that hurts, nothing else.

I think this passage describes the situation exactly, and not just in my exercise class. What matters is whether we contract away from strong energy or open to it. When we are in emotional pain, do we feel it and resonate with it and inquire into it? Or do we turn away from it by deadening it with drink or food or distraction?

Heliotroping is the art of turning to greet and embrace the energy. It increases our vibrance immensely, for a good and simple reason. We often are deluded to think that there is a faucet marked Pain and a faucet marked Pleasure—this thinking-error misinforms us that our job in life is to crank open the Pleasure faucet and keep the other one shut tight. The truth is that it's not possible to turn one faucet on and the other one off, because there is only one faucet. It's marked Awareness, and the choice is always the same in every moment: Turn it on or off. Unfortunately, many of us don't learn the truth until too late.

Vibrance *increases* through each act of opening the flow of Awareness. Vibrance *decreases* through each act of turning off the flow of Awareness. In order to enhance vibrance from moment to moment, we need to cultivate the habit of turning toward the issues and feelings that are seeking our attention.

What are some of these issues and feelings? There is one issue that constituted the biggest difference I noticed in the vibrantly mature people I interviewed. Vibrant people tend to be comfortable acknowledging the fears associated with aging, particularly the fear of death. If you ask vibrant people if they have any fears of dying, they tend to say something like "Sure, who doesn't?" If you ask non-vibrant people if they have fears of dying, they'll smile and assure you they don't fear death at all. They'll often go on to tell you that their faith makes them fearless. However, if you interview them side-by-side with vibrant people, you would see that denial is the more likely explanation.

The vibrant person gets comfortable with the fear of death through exploring it carefully, not by sealing it off beneath a layer of denial. Vibrant people have a willingness to wonder about death and the coming of age. Their comfort comes not from holding beliefs about death, but through acknowledging and exploring the fears, griefs, and angers that flow through them as they opened the Awareness faucet. Non-vibrant people are conspicuous in their lack of willingness to wonder and explore. They are quick to tell you of their convictions, beliefs, and opinions.

The Dalai Lama is certainly one of the most vibrantly mature people I have ever met. Ask him if he feels fear and he will say, "Certainly." He will tell you that he feels anxiety, sadness, even anger. Yet he radiates compassion like no other person in my experience. His Buddhist approach has taught him to stay open to all feelings and to transcend them through letting them be rather than shutting them out. The Dalai Lama exudes an organic compassion that derives from embracing all feelings and giving them room to breathe.

A lot of people I've encountered in my therapy office have come to harm through adopting an attitude exactly opposite to the Dalai Lama's. They have attempted to force themselves to feel positive emotions—such as compassion, forgiveness, and happiness—over the top of unacknowledged and unexplored feelings such as anger, grief, and fear. They may feel an emotion they don't want to experience, such as anger. Rather than heliotroping to explore it, they shrink away from it by contracting. This process takes place so fast that it becomes virtually subliminal. After a while, the flinch of contraction becomes so habitual that we may say, "I'm not afraid of death" and think we're telling the truth. The cost of that false-front is high—vibrance disappears behind the mask.

The Third Element: Essencing

As we mature, we feel a pressure from within to rest more at home in our authentic selves. If we resist the pressure to discover and embrace our essence—who we truly are—we cannot help but lose our natural vibrance. The trend of life is toward wholeness and authenticity; to resist this force is to invite exhaustion.

Almost all of us become skilled at wearing masks, especially in the early stages of life. Sometimes we have to put on masks to hide certain types of feelings in our families of origin. We may be born into a family that doesn't permit anger or one that doesn't permit fear, sadness, or even happiness. Since all humans are born with the same basic emotional wiring, we may find that our survival and success in our given family depends on masking one or more of the emotions we're wired to feel.

My childhood obesity, for example, was a painful way of protecting myself from what must have been perceived by me as the greater pain of feeling the griefs, angers, and fears that swirled within and around me. I know for a fact that I didn't lose the weight and keep it off until into my twenties, when I also learned how to feel my emotions instead of sealing them out of my awareness.

There are plenty of other reasons we learn to wear masks, and none of those reasons should be considered "bad." Many of our masks serve to keep the machinery of polite social discourse working smoothly. Imagine a world in which everyone always told the truth about everything. A traffic cop might be chewing you out and writing you a ticket when suddenly he says, "I just realized I'm still mad at my wife for an argument we didn't finish this morning. Don't take my anger personally." A politician might suddenly say, "I just told you I didn't have sex with that woman, but I actually did. We had sex a bunch of times and it was great! I lied because I want you to keep liking me." Personally, I would like to live in such a world, but it apparently isn't to everyone's taste just yet.

At midlife, however, our social masks begin to become painfully tight. We want to know who we really are and how we really feel about things. We want to know who others really are and how they really feel. We want others to know the real "us." A while back I met a vibrant woman, 50, striding down the street. She gave me a big hello and a bright smile. Although she seemed vaguely familiar, I wasn't sure who she was or whether I knew her. She introduced herself, and my jaw dropped open.

The last time I saw her she was in my office for the first and only time. She was on anti-depressant medication as well as a range of painkillers for arthritis. She had come to see me to get a "second opinion," and I assumed from her disappearance after one session that my opinion had been too radical for her taste. It turned out she followed my suggestions so thoroughly that she hadn't had time to report back in for a year.

I had told her that it looked like she'd been working overtime for a long time to maintain some masks she hated wearing. She agreed, saying that she hated the mansion she'd just moved into. She was questioning whether she even wanted to continue being the wife of a bank president. When I pressed her on this, she said she'd been in a sham marriage for years. She and her husband maintained it for the kids and the social status. She told me she was desperate for creative expression, "something more than picking out bathroom fixtures and decorative tiles." She and her husband both quietly kept secret lovers, though both of them "sort of" knew the supposed secret.

I told her it was up to her to choose, but that I thought she was at a make-or-break choice-point. I quoted William James to her on the way to change your life: *Do it now. Do it flamboyantly. No exceptions.*

I told her to go home and think about what she wanted to do, saying that I would be happy to work with her but only on the condition that she treat her arthritis and depressions as symptoms of wearing masks. I told her: If she would not commit to a process of removing the masks and embracing her authentic self, she would be better off staying on the medications. I don't charge a fee for my initial interview, leaving both myself and my prospective client free of obligation until we've had a chance to look each other over. She never called me back, so I assumed she had chosen to stay on the medical path. That was the last I heard of her until that day on the street.

The way she came bouncing down the sidewalk told me she was either off the anti-depressants or had found one that made me want some myself. The news was good: She said she was pain-free and medication-free. Then she told me the story, which made my step bouncy after we parted. After our session, she'd decided she was going to prove to herself that she had the power and the will to do her make-over herself. She flushed the painkillers down the toilet and started doing yoga three days a week. She told her husband she wanted to sell the house and get something simpler. She told him about her affairs and made herself available to hear the truth from him. They sent the kids to the grandparents for two weeks and went camping with nothing but a pup tent, supplies, and a couple of sleeping bags. There, in the heart of the forest, they found the heart of their marriage again. They committed themselves to living in a way that was free of the masks that separated them. They made vows to themselves and each other to discover their true selves and live their lives in harmony with who they really were.

And there she was, standing before me, with no arthritis and no depression. She and her husband had just returned from a week's volunteer labor for Habitat for Humanity, and she held out a calloused hand for me to shake in farewell. I watched her walk away, admiring that springy step again, and I felt a surge of hope. Here was a person who had chosen the unknown over the known, and it had worked out marvelously well. She knew how to wear her masks—we all know that so well—but she had opted for the exhilarating but potentially scary thrill ride of inventing a new and authentic self. None of us knows if we will like that new self or whether it will be acceptable to those around us. Here, though, was proof that it was not only possible but profoundly healthful.

I was much more than impressed—I was moved.

The Fourth Element: Innovating

We all have our routines: The way we drive to work, the sequence of our morning's self-care activities, the favorite snack at that certain time of the evening. These practiced moves give life a comfortable feel, a soothing sense of familiarity. Practice the same moves too long, though, and that comfortable, soothing feeling can become a numb, dumb trance.

Cultivating a vibrance-mindset involves acquiring a taste for innovation. Earlier in this chapter, when we discussed Flexing versus Sticking-to-Positions, we saw that some positions are worth sticking to but many are not. The same is true for routines and for the same reasons. Some routines serve our well-being and reflect values we've consciously chosen. However, many routines don't really contribute to well-being, and many others reflect no consciously chosen values at all.

For example, I meditate every morning and evening for 20 to 30 minutes. I haven't missed a day since 1973, so you could definitely call it part of my routine. It's one routine I have no intention of changing. Comparing my mood, my productivity, and my general health before '73 to the years since, my well-being has grown by quantum amounts. In addition, I value things like serenity, clarity, and daily deep communion with my spiritual essence—meditation provides all that and more. I chose those values. Nobody drilled them into me against my will or before I could think for myself.

Compare that routine with that of a fellow I met who'd eaten oatmeal every morning for thirty-four years. Perhaps you could make the case that his routine serves his well-being, but does it reflect values he's consciously chosen? Maybe, although I'm drawing a blank at the moment as to what those values might be. Let's give him the benefit of the doubt, though, and say that eating oatmeal serves his well-being and reflects his values.

Now, let's compare meditation and oatmeal with other routines, such as driving to work the same way every day or eating dinner at the same time each day. Neither of these routines serves well-being or reflects consciously chosen values. These latter examples are the kinds of routines that very much need our attention. Vibrant people look for ways to shake themselves out of the trance of numbing routine. They look for new ways to get to work. They eat at different times of the day, if for no other reason than to bust up an unnecessary pattern. If they catch themselves doing the same thing the same way for a few times in a row, they give themselves a wake-up call. By so doing, they keep the occasional routine from turning into a rut.

The vibrance-mindset is formed by making vibrant choices in tiny moments over time. If you pay close attention you will notice dozens of choice-moments throughout the day. One situation after another occurs in which we choose between Either's and Or's that carry profound consequences.

> Either we become more flexible or we harden into
> positions.
> Either we embrace experiences or we cringe away from
> them in contraction.
> Either we reveal our true selves or we hide behind
> masks.
> Either we renew ourselves through innovation or we cut
> a deeper groove into the rut of routine.

The richness and variety of human experience means that today—this day—right now—we will have opportunities galore to re-invent ourselves as the vibrant people we were born to be.

Achieving Vibrance

One simple way to begin—perhaps indeed the easiest—is to increase our flexibility in the physical realm, using an innovative movement that has brightened my day for years.

Turn the page and let me introduce you to a miracle you can create for yourself any time you want.

CHAPTER FOUR

Vibrant Physical Energy
The Most Important Two Minutes
of Your Vibrant Day

≋≋≋

THE MOST IMPORTANT SINGLE THING you can do to feel vibrant
each day is to create more flexibility in your spine. In other
words, if you want to wake up feeling better tomorrow than you
did today, your most effective action is two minutes of flexing
your spine in a certain way. In this chapter, you'll learn a unique
way of flexing that's so easy you can do it in your favorite chair or
even in bed. We call it the Vibrance-Flex. I want to inspire, beg,
and implore you to do a little bit of it each day. It changed my
life, and I am confident it will do the same for you.

> If your spine is flexible, you're young no matter your age.
> If your spine is *not* flexible, you're old no matter
> your age.
> It's a simple as that.

The magic of the Vibrance-Flex comes from its simplicity and absolute reliability. The Vibrance-Flex rapidly enhances physical energy even in people who have neglected their bodies for years. Practice it for as little as two minutes, preferably in the morning, and you feel a glow of well-being and mental clarity that stays with you all day.

After doing the Vibrance-Flex for a year or so I found that I could predict how I was going to feel based on how much of it I'd done that morning. Sometimes I was in a hurry and just did my two-minute "basic" program of the Flex. I would certainly feel good and definitely more energetic than before I discovered its magic. If I had time to do five minutes of the Flex, I would feel even more vital energy throughout the day. However, if I could devote ten minutes to doing the whole Vibrance-Flex series . . . Wow! I would zip around all day with virtually limitless energy. If I started to flag a little, I'd just do a few seconds of it in my car or at my desk. Zoom!—I'd be back in the flow again.

As you can probably tell by now, I'm an enthusiastic practitioner and my own best customer. Nowadays, I begin and end my day with the Vibrance-Flex. It's also woven into every hour in between. This morning at sunrise you would have seen me out on my deck, doing the Vibrance-Flex in the fresh air. At this moment, I'm sitting on a chair, doing the seated version of the Vibrance-Flex as I work at my desk. (The seated version is a subtle movement that cannot be detected by another person, so you don't have to worry about looking silly if you do it in a public place.) I also do a minute or two more at night, usually just before I go to bed. I find that even a minute or so of it helps me get a sounder night of sleep. Earlier in my life, my back often felt stiff and painful when I woke up in the morning. I haven't had a twinge of back pain in the five years since I started doing my Vibrance-Flex movements. That seems like a miracle to me.

Take a moment right now to discover for yourself how good it feels.

The Vibrance-Flex duplicates the way your spine was moving even before you were born. Many people don't realize it, but our bodies are in a constant flux of movement the whole time of our gestation. Osteopathic physicians were saying this back in the nineteenth century, but the orthodox medical establishment didn't believe it (and there was no way to prove it until the ultrasound a hundred years later could verify it). I'll have more to say about the details later in this chapter.

If you're sitting up, here's how the Vibrance-Flex works: Gently arch and flatten the small of your back. If you're sitting in a chair, you can arch and flatten the small of your back against the back of the chair. Do it slowly, taking five or six seconds to arch, and the same amount of time to flatten the small of the back. Notice that when you arch the small of your back, your head naturally tilts upward, and as you flatten the small of your back, your head naturally tilts downward. The entire time of your gestation—from the time you were the size of a caterpillar to the moment of your birth—your spine was doing this movement, at about the same speed I've invited you to do it.

The movement continues after we're born. You can feel it

and see it easily in babies, but by the time we've been in school for a while the movement is harder to detect. Again, I'll explain a lot more about it later in the chapter, but for now, take a moment to enjoy this movement and to celebrate its profound effect on your well-being.

WHY THE VIBRANCE-FLEX WORKS SO WELL

Most of us think of ourselves as solid. From one perspective we certainly are. If you close your eyes for a moment as you walk down a crowded sidewalk, you'll quickly find out just how solid you are. Thinking of ourselves as solid comes in handy at times, especially when we want to feel stable, hard, and invincible. On the downside, there are problems with thinking of ourselves as solid. For one, solid objects are not very flexible, and flexibility is an important quality as we move through life. Solid objects also wear out: Even a big, hard thing like the Grand Canyon suffers from erosion over time. Meanwhile, the water just keeps on flowing.

The big problem with thinking of ourselves as solid is that we really aren't. We are more fluid than solid, more flowing than hard. Our bodies are a living river system, full of tributaries, gullies, and major waterways. Just as all rivers eventually come to the sea, our living river-system begins and ends in an ocean. Our brain, our spine—indeed, our whole identity—actually floats in an ocean, and that ocean even has tides in it.

Vibrant Physical Energy

The ocean we float in is called the cerebrospinal fluid. Our ancestors, the original life-forms, came from the ocean long ago. Now, we carry the descendant of that ocean around with us. It is a magnificent paradox: We carry the ocean within us, and the ocean carries us within it.

First, look at it on a purely physical level. There is an all-one-piece membrane around our brain and spine. Think of it as a cellophane wrapper around your brain and spine, extending from the top of your brain down to your tailbone. Within this wrapper is a living body of fluid that nurtures and nourishes the essential center of ourselves from brain to tailbone. Our brain and spine—the very center of who we are—float within that ocean every moment of our lives.

I was speaking literally, not metaphorically, when I said there are tides in the ocean we live in. The cerebrospinal fluid expands and recedes about every six seconds. You can feel these tides yourself. If you tune in sensitively to the cerebrospinal fluid, you can feel it expand and contract every six seconds or so. A simple way to do it is to rest your fingertips lightly on your head just above your ears. You'll probably need to hold your breath to feel the cerebrospinal movements, because breathing also causes expanding and contracting. Hold your breath for ten or fifteen seconds and see if you can feel your skull expanding and contracting every six seconds or so. I've taught hundreds of people to do this, and most of them have been able to feel it within a couple of minutes of tuning in.

Another way to feel your inner tide is to touch your tongue

lightly to the roof of your mouth. The tidal action of the cerebrospinal fluid causes the roof of your mouth to rise and fall
slightly every six seconds or so. At first you may not feel anything—it's a subtle movement—but once you feel it there's no
mistaking it. The tide is caused by the pumping of your cerebrospinal fluid, keeping your brain and spine bathed in a nurturing matrix that has been with you since before you were born. In
fact, part of the cerebrospinal system is called the *pia mater,*
which in Latin means the *soft mother.*

The Vibrance-Flex exercise I want you to do every morning
is designed to open more space for your inner-ocean to flow. Any
body of water is healthier when it flows and breathes. Opening up more space each day for your inner-ocean to move is
the number-one most important thing you can do for vibrance
each day.

WITNESSING MIRACLES

Many years ago, I was blessed to come into contact with a gifted
osteopathic physician, Dr. Viola Frymann. When I met her, Dr.
Frymann was well into her sixties, although she had the energy
and stamina of a teenager.

Spending one day watching her work in her clinic was
enough to make me a true believer. Let me describe the first
thing I witnessed. Her first patient was a colicky infant who,
according to her mother, had been screaming non-stop for a
week. Understandably, the mother was at her wit's end. I don't

think I've ever seen a human being look so frazzled. My nerves were soon on edge, too—just a couple of minutes of the baby's harrowing shrieks was enough to do it.

Without a word, Dr. Frymann took the baby in her arms and held it for ten seconds or so. Then she cradled the baby's neck and head in one hand and began the treatment. Within less than a minute, the baby's screams subsided to whimpers. A minute later, the baby was sound asleep in Dr. Frymann's arms. At the moment the baby fell asleep, her mother collapsed in sobs in a chair. All I could do was bow my head: I felt that I was in the presence of the sacred, having witnessed a real miracle by the touch of a true angel.

Dr. Frymann was quick to point out, however, in her clipped accent and no-nonsense manner, that it was pure science. She did it all day long. Indeed, I watched her do it all day—with teenagers, with elders, with more babies. Sometimes the treatment took twenty minutes rather than two, but one person after the other walked out of the office with smiles on their faces. By the end of the day, I was not only deeply impressed, I was very keen on learning her secret.

Her secret, which she had learned from her teacher, Dr. William Sutherland, was that a certain movement occurs in our bodies from the moment we're conceived. The purpose of the movement is to circulate the all-important cerebrospinal fluid around the brain and spine. Osteopathic physicians called it the "craniosacral pulsation," because it involved a complex set of interactions from the sacrum all the way up into the bones of the cranium. The Vibrance-Flex activity I want you to do every morning is based on these very same organic movements.

STRESSES AND TRAUMAS

The craniosacral pulsation is sensitive, but it's also very resilient. Life's traumas shut it down, and the hindered movement affects our moods, our health, our energy-level. However, with the proper exercise or the gifted hands of a healer, it can be restored to its natural movement fairly quickly. Dr. Sutherland developed a healing system for unwinding the kinks left by trauma. By certain hands-on techniques he discovered and refined, the craniosacral pulsation could be set free again. Dr. Frymann had learned it from him and passed it along to another generation of her fellow-physicians.

Dr. Frymann and her colleagues were interested in using the hands-on manipulations as a medical treatment. However, I was interested in *preventive* procedures. As I studied the craniosacral pulsation, I began to see possibilities that extended far outside the consulting room. Not everyone has access to gifted healing hands—I sought something we could do for ourselves each day as a self-help tool. So, in consultation with Dr. Frymann and other colleagues, I developed a set of gentle flexes that re-awakened and restored the craniosacral pulsation on a daily basis. My exercises put the movement into play in its ideal form, just as it was before life's traumas jammed it up.

Dr. Frymann was very generous with sharing her secrets

with me and hundreds of other colleagues. I will gladly share my "secret" with anyone within shouting distance: Start your day with a few minutes of the Vibrance-Flex. Then, throughout the day, whenever you become aware that you don't feel energetic and harmonious, do a few Vibrance-Flexes right on the spot. If you're sitting down, do the seated version. You can do it in the seat of your car or your box seat at Yankee Stadium. If you're walking down the street, do the walking version. If you're lying down, do the lying-down version.

I think you get the idea—you can do it anywhere.

WHAT IT LOOKS LIKE

Here are pictures of the basic Vibrance-Flex. These will show you how your body should move when you do the Vibrance-Flex.

We'll begin with the seated Vibrance-Flex, the first activity in your daily Vibrance program.

1. Sit upright . . . gently arch and flatten the small of your back . . . as you arch your head tilts up and as you flatten the small of your back your head tilts down . . . Do that a few times, keeping it slow and gentle.

2. Notice any places in the movement where you feel stiff. When you come to those gritchy places, slow down and go very gently through them. If you encounter pain or unpleas-

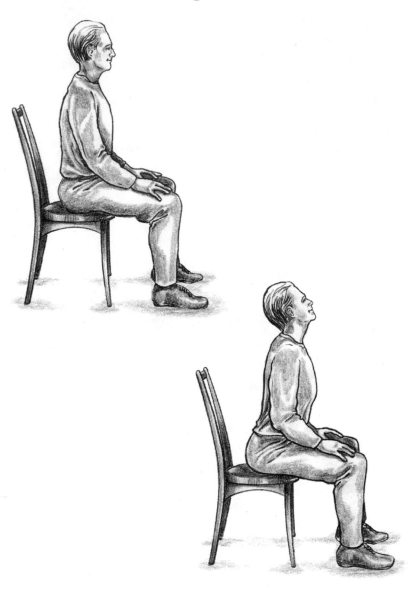

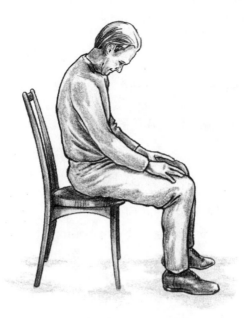

ant tension, pause or make the movement very small so that you don't hurt or feel unpleasant sensations.

3. After a minute or so, pause and rest and notice your body sensations.

4. After you've rested for a moment, begin again . . . gently arch and flatten the lower part of the back, tuning in now to both the small of your back up to the middle between your shoulder-blades. Let that whole area participate . . . as you arch look up toward the ceiling and as you flatten look down

toward the floor. Keep your neck relaxed with no strain or buckling. Flex slowly, taking 6 seconds to go in one direction and 6 seconds to go in the other.

5. Now pause and rest and tune in to your body-sensations.

6. Notice anything that's different than when we began.

HOW TO PRACTICE AT HOME

Pick a time of day that's good for you. Most people like to do it first-thing in the morning, but that's completely up to you. Do the Flex for a minute, then rest for a few seconds. Do another minute and then rest. After two to four rounds, most people are feeling more energy and well-being. You can do several sessions a day. Always remember to do it slow and easy and in the comfort zone. Do your best to do it every day. Most people feel a noticeable different right away, but I predict you'll start feeling really good after you've done the Flex reliably for a few days.

HOW TO COORDINATE YOUR BREATHING WITH THE VIBRANCE-FLEX

Your breathing is designed to work in harmony with the movement of the Vibrance-Flex. In fact, learning how to link up your breathing with the Vibrance-Flex could be the most important thing you ever do to feel good all day long. This is especially true if you have ever had the common problems of breathing that many people have—problems such as feeling short of breath, yawning, feeling like you can never quite get a full breath.

When I first became interested in breathing over thirty years ago, I set myself the task of watching a hundred babies breathe. I wanted to find out from these "experts" what breathing looked like in its natural state, before life's traumas interfered with the delicate mechanisms of the breath. By watching babies breathe, then comparing what I saw with observations of elementary and high-school students, I got a very practical education in what goes wrong with our breathing and how we can set it right again.

If you watch a healthy baby breathe, you will see that it breathes in harmony with the movement of the Vibrance-Flex. In other words, the baby moves its spine slightly with every breath, and it does so in exactly the same movement as you learned earlier. This is the healthy breathing pattern of babies (and adults, too):

- When the baby breathes in, the small of the back arches slightly and the head tilts up.

- When the baby breathes out, the small of the back flattens and the head tilts down.

- The baby "belly-breathes." The in-breath causes the belly to round, and the out-breath causes the belly to flatten.

However—and this is very important—*the coordination of breath and movement disappears when the baby becomes distressed.* In fact, the healthy pattern not only disappears, it often turns upside-down and backward:

- Under distress, the baby's belly tenses, forcing the breath up into the chest. The baby stops "belly-breathing" and takes shorter, shallower breaths up in the chest. This is the opposite of the healthy pattern.

- Under distress, the harmony of spine-and-breath movement disappears. Sometimes the movement will be the reverse of the healthy pattern, with the in-breath coming in coordination with the flattening of the small of the back, as though the breath is fighting with the movement. At other times, the pattern is simply no pattern at all—chaotic movements that have no observable relationship to each other.

When the stress is relieved, the baby goes back to breathing in harmony with the Vibrance-Flex movement of the spine.

Now that you understand how this works, and why it's so important, let's take a few minutes to try it on in your body.

Here is a picture of how your breathing is designed to link up with the movements of your spine.

1. Sit upright, with your back a few inches away from the seat-back so that it has room to move.

2. Gently, slowly arch and flatten the small of your back. When you flatten the small of your back, move as if you were going to press the small of your back against the seat-back; when you arch the small of your back, move as if you were going to arch away from the seat-back. Do this very slowly and gently. Make the movement as big as you comfortably can. Remember, though, in this and every other activity in this book: Never strain—always stay in the zone of ease.

3. When you feel at ease with this simple arching-and-flattening movement, continue doing it as you add another dimension. Notice, as you arch and flatten the small of your back, that your head and chin tilts upward as you arch and downward as you flatten.

4. Tune in sensitively to your spine, feeling how the movement of your head is intimately connected to the movement of your lower back. Feel the simple elegance of this movement.

5. As you arch the small of your back, take a full, easy in-breath. As you flatten the small of your back, take a full, easy out-breath.

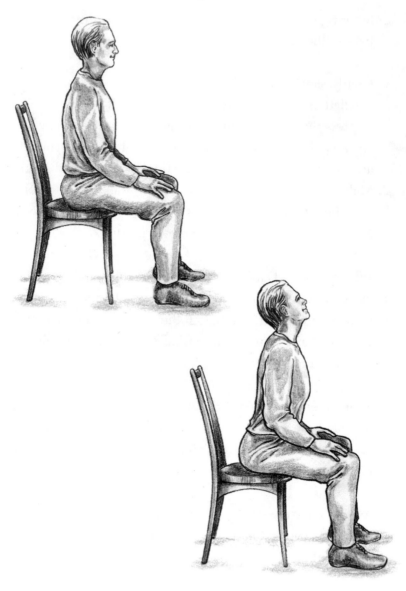

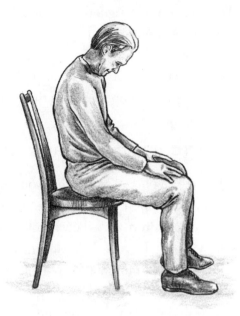

6. As you breathe in, arching the small of your back, relax the muscles of your belly so that the breath seems to fill and round your belly.

7. As you breathe out, flattening the small of your back, let your belly flatten at the same time.

8. As you breathe in, let your head and chin tilt upward as your back arches and your belly rounds.

9. As you breathe out, let your head and chin tilt downward as your back and belly flatten.

This is the way nature designed your breathing to work in harmony with the movement of your spine.

Breathe this way for a minute or two, keeping the breath slow, deep, and easy while at the same time arching and flattening the small of your back in harmony with the breath.

RECOGNIZING THE DISTRESS PATTERN

Let's explore the pattern of distress, so that you can recognize it when it happens. And happen it will—almost every person will experience the distress pattern on a daily if not hourly basis. The trick to life is not avoiding distress—it's knowing how to handle it and how to return to a harmonious body-feeling as quickly as possible. In other words, you won't always be able to avoid your boss or someone else getting mad at you, but you can learn how to get back to feeling centered quickly after the person has stormed out the door.

Re-Creating the Distress Pattern

Let's re-create the distress pattern in slow motion, so that you can get a whole-body picture of how it affects you.

1. Begin by creating healthy, natural movement and breathing.

2. Sit upright, and begin to arch and flatten the small of your back slowly and gently. As you arch the small of your back,

let your head and chin tilt up, and as you flatten the small of your back let your head and chin tilt down.

3. As you arch the small of your back, take a full belly-breath in. As you flatten the small of your back, take a full belly-breath out.

4. Do a few cycles of this, keeping it slow and easy.

5. Now, create the distress pattern. When something distressful happens, your stomach muscles tighten. Tense your belly-muscles now, and keep them tight as you arch and flatten the small of your back. Keep them tense as you try to take a full belly-breath. Feel how even a little bit of tension in your stomach muscles affects your movement and your breathing.

6. Relax your stomach muscles now, and do a few cycles of healthy, natural breathing and moving. Take full belly-breaths as you arch and flatten the small of your back.

7. Now let's add more of the distress pattern. When something distressful happens, not only do your stomach muscles harden, but you also clench your jaw and take shallower breaths higher up in your chest. Your breathing shifts from belly to chest.

8. Harden your stomach muscles while clenching your jaw at the same time. Take shallow breaths in your high chest while you continue to keep your stomach muscles tight. Feel how this affects your movements and breathing.

9. Now, relax everything and go back to natural, healthy breathing and moving. Arch and flatten the small of your back, taking a full belly-breath in as you arch and a full belly-breath out as you flatten.

THE STANDING VIBRANCE-FLEX

The Vibrance-Flex works wonders when done in a standing position, too. In fact, since you have more stretching capabilities from a standing position, you'll probably get an even stronger sense of vibrance from the standing version of the V-Flex.

1. Stand with your feet hip-width and your arms relaxed at your sides. Arch and flatten the small of your back, taking three to four seconds to arch and three to four seconds to flatten.

2. As you arch, look up toward the ceiling, and when you flatten, look down toward the floor. Keep the back of your neck relaxed as you look up and down. As you arch and look up, feel your chest widen, and when you flatten your back and look down, feel your chest narrow. Breathe in fully as you arch and look up, then breathe out fully as you flatten and

look down. Keep your breathing slow and easy, taking at least three to four seconds to breathe in and three to four seconds to breathe out.

3. After thirty seconds or so, pause and rest for a little while.

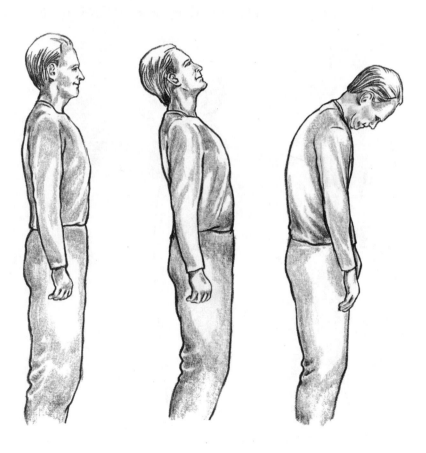

1. For the next part of the standing V-Flex, raise your arms in front of you.

2. Begin as you did before—arching and flattening the small of your back as you look up and down. This time, widen your arms as you arch and look up, then close your arms over your chest as if you're embracing yourself tightly as you flatten

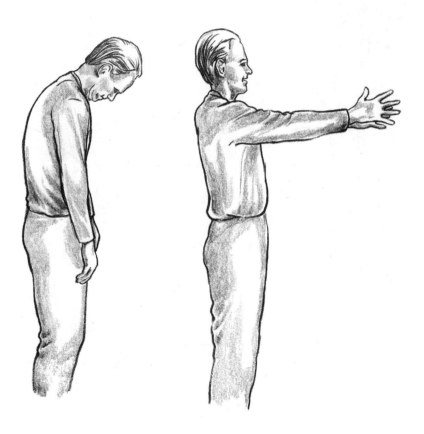

and look down. Breathe in as you open your arms wide, and breathe out as you close your arms over your chest.

3. After a few cycles, pause and rest with your arms at your sides.

4. When you're ready to continue, raise your arms again in front of you. This time, raise your arms toward the ceiling as you arch, breathe in and look up, then sweep your arms down toward the floor as you breathe out. Go as far down as you feel comfortable. It's not a contest, so stay in your comfort zone.

5. As soon as you've finished your out-breath, breathe in as you straighten back up, reaching your arms toward the ceiling. Do this slowly, taking at least three to four seconds to breathe in and three to four seconds to breathe out. Continue for thirty seconds or so, then pause to rest.

The Origins of the Vibrance-Flex

Where did the Vibrance-Flex originate? The craniosacral pulsation—the organic movements the Vibrance-Flex is based on—began long before any of us were aware of it. In fact, it was going on even before we were born! While you were inside your mother's womb, your fetal body was doing the Vibrance-Flex. Watch an ultrasound closely and you can see it plain as day.

After we're born, the Vibrance-Flex continues throughout

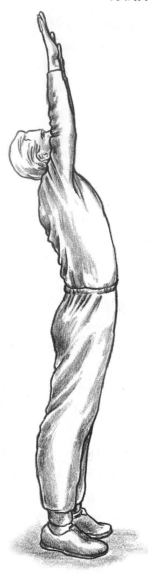
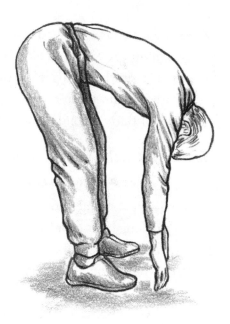

our nursing and bonding time of the first year of life. I've felt its gentle elongation-and-contraction in dozens of babies I've held. I've watched it in hundreds more. The Vibrance-Flex is essential to life, and it continues throughout life.

However—and this is a very big, important however—this essential movement can be jostled, jammed, and compromised by the stresses and traumas of life. I've had trouble seeing and feeling it in people who have been traumatized by a wide variety of life-events:

- People who have been in collisions, such as car and bike accidents.

- Athletes who have slammed their bodies against something, whether through tackling, falling down, being hit, or other shocks.

- Children and adults who have been physically abused.

- Children and adults who have been emotionally abused, especially those who have been criticized a lot.

- Adults who sit too much without moving.

These and other stressors put crimps in the elegance and ease of the Vibrance-Flex. That's why it's so important to take two minutes each day *to revive it and re-create it in its ideal form.*

When you do the Vibrance-Flex each morning, you bring it to life again in its perfect form. In other words, you re-conceive yourself in your most fundamental way. Remember, the movement has been with you since your conception. When you do it according to the instructions I give you, you return yourself to the beginning and get a fresh start. The Vibrance-Flex exercises re-create the natural movement. Take a couple of minutes a day to do the Vibrance-Flex—just as nature intended your spine to move—and you'll recover your birthright of a vibrant flow of energy throughout the day.

CREATING A PROGRAM FOR YOURSELF

As I mentioned earlier, I found that I could predict how vibrant I felt all day by how much of the V-Flex I did in the morning. Two minutes of it gives me a "maintenance" level of vibrance. Five minutes gives me a much zippier feeling all day. If I take the time to do the full series, I feel such a powerful sense of vibrance streaming through me all day that it still surprises me.

Since it feels so good, you might think I'd take time to do the full ten minutes of the Basic and Advanced V-Flex every day. However, I don't. Often I get caught up in the same kinds of situations you probably do. I get a late start, or I get a phone call, or there's a meeting I need to get to. Counting up over the past year, I probably get the full series in a few times a week. The majority of the time, though, I do at least my "maintenance" dose and often a few of the Advanced Flexes.

Vibrant Physical Energy

Later in the book you'll see that I've created two different programs:

- The Seven-Minute Foundation Program
- The Advanced Program

The Seven-Minute Program includes two minutes of the V-Flex activities combined with the other elements of the program. The Advanced Program includes the full V-Flex series.

I encourage you to try them both out several times so that you're familiar with how they make you feel. If you have time (and if you can stand feeling that good!), I recommend the Advanced Program. I've personally taught it to thousands of people, so I've had an up-close opportunity to see the miracles it can work. However, the Seven-Minute Foundation Program has all the absolute essentials in it. It's simply a matter of how good we want to feel.

That brings us to another mention of something we've touched on before: the nearly-universal resistance to feeling really good. My wife and I first noticed it in our own relationship as well as in relationship therapy. We started calling it the Upper Limits Problem, because it was as if we had a "governor" on our feel-good thermostat. Once a certain level of good feeling had been exceeded, we would automatically do something to bring ourselves back down. We would be feeling really good, then one of us would make a criticism or a joke or bring up a household issue. Poof!—the flow of positive energy would disappear.

101

Be prepared to confront the Upper Limits Problem when you start doing the Vibrance-Flex and other elements of the program. The program makes you feel good, and it does it quickly. Sometimes the program makes people feel better than they've ever felt in their lives. We've had many people come back with a report that goes something like this: "I did the program for a couple of days and I felt really great. Then, next time I thought about it, I realized I hadn't done it for a week."

That's the Upper Limits Problem at work. Part of us wants to feel great, but another part of us wants to keep things exactly the way they are, even if the way we are is not so good. Why? Because part of the mind is focused exclusively on survival. This older, more primitive part of the mind thinks: I felt awful yesterday and I survived, so maybe I did something right. Let's feel awful again today! If we start feeling really good, let's arrange for something to happen to make us feel awful again!

Another part of our mind is focused on higher things: creativity, innovation, enlightenment, feeling great. However, as yet human beings do not have as much experience with feeling enlightened or vibrant or creative as we do with suffering. Suffering comes very naturally to us—we've had a great deal of practice at it.

That's why I caution you to expect the Upper Limits Problem as you begin to do the Vibrance program. You'll feel more vibrant, and it may be more vibrance than you're accustomed to. Expect that you'll set yourself back more than once. You'll suddenly "forget" to do the program or you'll "forget" where you put your book. You'll "get too busy" or you'll hurt your back playing golf so you "can't" do the program. In my notes I've recorded several hundred variations of each of those moves. They all boil down to the Upper Limits Problem, our eternal wrestling match with whether we deserve to feel great all the time.

When the Upper Limit Problem occurs, just remember that it's natural and normal and no big deal. As soon as you spot it, there's only one move that matters: Re-commit to feeling vibrant. Then turn to the page with the program on it and spend ten or twenty minutes opening up to the stream of vibrance again. With patience and practice, you'll become accustomed to vibrance.

Speaking personally, I can tell you it's well worth the investment of time and energy. It's been years now since I've felt anything but great. It took a couple of years of daily practice to get vibrance as an "always-on" feeling that doesn't fade. I don't mind that it took ten or twenty minutes a day to make that possible.

If I'm enjoying a journey with my car humming along smoothly, I don't mind the hour I spent getting my oil changed that morning. In fact, I take pride in taking good care of what I've been blessed with. That's how I feel about the Vibrance-Flex.

Living in a human bodymind is like inheriting the Taj Mahal. Maintaining it is a way of honoring the gift.

I inherited the great gift of a human bodymind, as did you.

Let's honor that blessing by opening the windows of our own private Taj each day to let the breeze blow through. Let's commit a few minutes of our day to letting the flow of vibrance stream through us.

Enjoying the breeze and honoring the gift: Until I can think of a better meaning of life, I'm going to go with that one.

CHAPTER FIVE

Breathing for Vibrance

To FEEL GOOD is to breathe well. To breathe well is to feel good.

The evidence is clear, however, that most of us don't feel as good as we could simply because we don't breathe well. I've seen scientific research indicating that as many as four out of every five adults don't breathe well. My clinical experience confirms these studies. Most people I've worked with have benefited enormously from even a little bit of attention to their breathing. Indeed, a little bit of attention is usually all it takes to learn to breathe well. A good breath is a high-leverage investment—you multiply it times twenty thousand every day.

Breathing seems like such a simple thing to do, but most of us don't know the simple secrets to making it easy. For nearly three decades I've been a student and teacher of breathing, yet almost every day I find another subtle, tiny improvement I can make in my breathing. I've witnessed miracle after miracle in the lives of my clients as they've learned to make the tiny corrections that lead to healthy breathing.

A PERSONAL BREAKTHROUGH

I don't think I paid a second's attention to my breathing until one magic moment when I was in my twenties. I was fresh out of my Ph.D. program, and like a lot of newly minted Ph.D.'s, I thought I knew just about all there was to know about just about everything. One day I found out how little I knew about something incredibly important. The discovery changed my life.

A gifted holistic doctor, Jack Downing, M.D., took a look at me and said, "Dr. Hendricks, you're never going to feel good if you keep breathing like that." He showed me what I was doing wrong, and he assured me that my breathing problems were very common. In less than an hour, he taught me how to breathe effectively.

I'll never forget those first moments of being able to breathe the way nature intended. When I opened up to my full breathing capacity I felt a miraculous shift inside me—bliss surged through me in wave after wave. My mood brightened, fatigue disappeared, and chronic pain melted from my neck and shoulders. All my life I'd felt slightly tired and off-center. I didn't think there was anything unusual about that off-center feeling—in fact, that was the way I thought everybody felt. All that time I'd only been a few good breaths away from feeling good!

≋

Our breathing is exquisitely sensitive. Many things disturb it—accidents, tensions in your daily life, emotional problems like getting criticized. Under stress, your breathing shifts into fight-or-flight mode. If you don't know how to recover your natural breathing, you'll feel tired or moody just because of the way you breathe. A small correction can bring a delicious feeling of ease within seconds. A few natural breaths can even turn emotions like anger or fear into pleasant waves of energy. Thirty years of solid scientific research has proven that natural breathing helps everything from public-speaking anxiety to insomnia.

WHAT IT TAKES

There are three specific errors the majority of people make in their breathing. I lump them together and call them by one name: the Central Breathing Problem. I think of it as one problem because most people do all three things wrong at the same time. In a nutshell, here's what causes most of our problems with breathing:

- We breathe too shallow.
- We breathe too fast.
- We breathe upside-down.

The obvious solution is to breathe slower, deeper, and right-side-up. There's an art to learning how to do that, and I want you to master that art by practicing the simple suggestions in this chapter.

It's easy to understand what it means to breathe too shallow and too fast. However, upside-down breathing may need some explanation (for example, it doesn't mean we breathe standing on our heads!).

The best way to understand healthy breathing is to watch a healthy baby breathe. When it breathes in, its belly rises and rounds. The baby's belly-muscles stay relaxed, so that the breath can get deep down into the bottom of its lungs. When you see an unhealthy adult breathe, the exact opposite occurs (which is why we call it upside-down breathing). Most adults hold their belly muscles too tightly. The belly-tension keeps the lungs from expanding fully.

Imagine wearing a tight girdle around your middle. When your breath comes in, the expansion of your lungs comes up against the immovable wall of the belly. The belly can't relax and round, so the lungs cannot expand to their fullest.

Something has to give. What happens is that the girdle-around-the-middle causes the breath to be forced up into the chest, inflating it to accommodate the pressure. When you breathe high in your chest you must take short, shallow breaths at a faster rate, as opposed to the slower, deeper breathing that occurs when you keep your belly relaxed.

In the extreme, this breathing problem is associated with

high blood pressure, asthma, and other respiratory diseases. Fortunately, most of us don't have the problem to the extent that we need medical treatment, but almost all of us have the problem to a certain degree. Why? The reason is very simple: because we live in the twenty-first century!

Those of us who live in modern, urban environments are likely to have at least a mild version of the problem. By contrast, I've pedalled my bike across Tibet, where one would expect the high altitudes to cause rampant breathing problems. However, I never saw a single person with the Central Breathing Problem. Even though they were at 14,000 feet, the people were breathing slow, deep, and right-side-up. The problem is definitely not caused by a shortage of oxygen.

What's the problem, then? Why do four out of five people in Manhattan or Los Angeles have the Central Breathing Problem, while their thin-air Tibetan cousins don't? There are two main reasons: emotional stress and air pollution. The background noise of cities is the soundtrack to a disaster movie: sirens, jackhammers, honking horns, screeching brakes, people shouting over the din. This alone is enough to keep us in fight-or-flight mode. Then, factor in the emotional "noise" that pervades life—criticism, money struggles, family stresses. Finally, stir in a generous admixture of air pollution, and you have a pungent and potent atmosphere for bad breathing.

When life first evolved, the oxygen content of the air was over thirty percent. Nowadays, even in ideal settings such as redwood forests and country glens, the oxygen content of the air is

around twenty-three percent. In the urban canyons of Manhattan or freeway-ribboned L.A., the oxygen content is below 20
percent, with a nearly constant haze caused by exhaust fumes
and dust.

I had never seen smog before I first came to Los Angeles in
the early seventies. The first day, I was taking a walk with a friend
who'd lived there for several years. I pointed off toward the tall
buildings in the distance, semi-shrouded by a thick layer of
smog. "Look how smoggy it is over there," I said. My friend
smiled at my naïve observation. "And they're over there, point-
ing at us, saying how smoggy it is over here." Since I couldn't see
the smog in front of my eyes or feel it going up my nose, I
thought it was "over there."

What the Central Breathing Problem Feels Like

When we breathe too fast and too shallow, we discharge
more carbon dioxide than we should. Our bodies are designed to
operate in a very narrow range of oxygen/carbon dioxide balance. It doesn't take much shallow, rapid breathing to throw off
the balance. When the balance goes off-kilter, our bodies go into
a mild state of alarm.

You feel several specific sensations when your "breathing
chemistry" is out of balance:

- A little tired all the time, even when you first wake up.
- A little anxious, even though you may not be able to point
  to anything scary in your environment.

- Like you never quite get a full breath.
- Mental fog.

The Central Breathing Problem can usually be remedied fairly quickly. Most people I've worked with can get the basics in under an hour, and many can do it themselves by following simple self-help instructions. It's an endeavor well worth the time— you feel an immediate sense of ease and well-being the moment you get your breathing balanced.

HOW A HEALTHY DEEP BREATH LOOKS AND FEELS

I've been asked one question about breathing more than any other: *What does a correct breath actually look and feel like?*

The best way to understand a healthy deep breath is first to know what it isn't. When a doctor, stethoscope in hand, asks people to "take a deep breath," they often inflate their chests in an exaggerated way. While this move is adequate for giving doctors the information they need, it is absolutely the wrong way to breathe for good health.

A healthy deep in-breath occurs in three stages: Beginning, middle, and peak. A healthy deep out-breath goes through those three stages in reverse.

The In-Breath

Begin by relaxing the belly muscles. This allows the diaphragm to flatten and draw in the air. Your abdomen expands first, before your chest moves, which allows air to fill the lower part of your lungs.

The middle of the in-breath expands the chest muscles, which causes the rib cage to widen in three dimensions: front, side, and back. Your rib cage also moves upward as the air fills the middle part of your lungs.

At the peak of the in-breath, your collarbones move upward and your shoulders relax and move back slightly. Air fills the upper part of the lungs.

The Out-Breath

At the beginning of the out-breath, your collarbones drop and your shoulders move slightly forward.

In the middle of the out-breath, chest muscles relax as the rib cage moves downward and narrows in three dimensions.

At the end of the out-breath, the abdomen flattens and the belly muscles contract slightly.

By no means do I recommend that you pay attention to this level of detail with every breath. However, I've found that most people can benefit from a few minutes of "slow-motion" attention to all phases on an in-breath and out-breath, in order to map out the territory of a healthy breath. The most common mistake with breathing is to keep the belly muscles too tight, so that the diaphragm cannot flatten and move downward to allow a full in-breath. If this one problem can be solved, your breathing will increase in efficiency dramatically.

OXYGEN BALANCE

Your body is designed to function best at a specific and precise oxygen/CO_2 ratio. I call this ideal ratio the "oxygen balance-point" or "O-Balance." As I mentioned before, our sensitive breathing mechanism is affected by things like air pollution, accidents, stress, and tension. Under stress, people breathe too fast and too shallow, as well as throwing their breathing upside-down by tensing muscles that should stay relaxed during breath-ing. This learned habit throws off your O-Balance.

The symptoms of oxygen imbalance—chronic fatigue, anxi-ety, difficulty sleeping—are so common that many think it's nor-mal to experience them. I predict that you'll be surprised and pleased to find how easy it is to re-balance your breathing. After a few days of practice, most of our participants report that what they thought was "normal" was just due to poor breathing habits.

Suddenly, it becomes normal to feel:

- Mental clarity instead of fog.
- Harmony instead of background-noise anxiety.
- Pep instead of fatigue.
- The sense that your breathing is rich and full—your friend rather than your enemy.

It all depends on you, of course. It's your willingness to do the work (even though it's work that's easy and feels good) that makes it happen. I urge you to take a few minutes each day to bring your breathing back into balance. Once you do, you'll seldom have to think about it again. It will be your friend for life, nurturing you twenty thousand times a day with harmony, clarity, and ease.

THE VIBRANCE-BREATH: HOW TO MAINTAIN IDEAL OXYGEN BALANCE

In the last chapter, when you were learning the Vibrance-Flex, you also learned how to coordinate your breathing with the movements of your spine. This is essential to good health. Now, as we turn our attention to the Vibrance-Breath, keep in mind what you've learned about breathing in harmony with the movement of your spine. In fact, I will remind you of it now and then as we go through the instructions for the Vibrance-Breath.

You only need to practice the Vibrance-Breath a few minutes each day. Ideally, practice it a few minutes in the morning as part of your Daily Vibrance Program (details for the 10-minute version and the 20-minute advanced version appear later in the book). Once your body learns to recognize the good feelings caused by the Vibrance-Breath, it gravitates toward staying in balance all by itself.

The Vibrance-Breath: Beginning Instructions

You're going to learn a gentle breathing activity that's designed to help you feel more relaxed, alert, and clear. If you do it gently and correctly, after a minute or two you'll feel much clearer in your mind and at ease in your body. It's easy to learn—the only thing you have to remember is to do it comfortably with no strain or stressful effort.

Begin with a few cycles of the Vibrance-Flex, breathing in harmony with your body movements (as you learned in the last chapter).

The Vibrance-Breath re-balances the oxygen ratio in your body. In a moment, I'll ask you to breathe all your air out, then pause with all the air out of your body until your body really needs to breathe in again. This is not a contest, so don't strain in any way. As you do the Vibrance-Breath, you'll probably notice that you can go longer and longer without needing to breathe in. When your oxygen is perfectly balanced with the carbon dioxide in your body, you can go for a minute or so without needing to breathe in. In the early stages, though, you may only be able to go for a few seconds without needing to breathe in. That's why I say it's not a contest. Above all, don't strain or try too hard. This activity is always done in the comfort zone. You'll know when your oxygen balance–point is reached because you'll feel a sense of harmony and well-being. Until you feel that sensation, just practice in a gentle, comfortable way. Before you begin, scan

Achieving Vibrance

your body and notice if you feel tired or mentally foggy or any nervousness. After you do a minute or so of the Vibrance-Breath, I'll ask you to scan your body again and notice any changes in your body and mind.

Now, if you're ready, let's begin. On your next out-breath, breathe all the way out, then pause and relax until your body gives you a clear signal that it needs to breathe. It doesn't matter if you pause two seconds or 20 seconds before you breathe in. Just pause and relax until you get that clear signal that it's time to breathe in. Then take a full in-breath, as much as is comfortable. Then breathe all your breath out again and wait until you get a clear signal to breathe in. Do a few cycles now, then pause after about a minute. (Practice for a minute.)

As you rest, scan your body again. Notice if there is any change in sensations such as fatigue, nervousness, or lack of mental clarity. Some people feel positive shifts right away, while others take more practice before they notice changes.

Next time you breathe out, keep on breathing out until all the air is gone, then pause and relax before you let any back in. It's not important whether you wait a second or 30 seconds . . . just relax until you get a clear signal that your body needs to breathe. You may feel a few little false signals that you need to breathe in, but wait until your body spontaneously says "time to breathe." Then let an in-breath come all the way in and then breathe all the way out again. After you've breathed out, pause and relax until you get a clear signal that your body needs the next breath. Then breathe all the way in—as much as you like—

then breathe it all out, pause, and relax. Practice for a couple of minutes now, remembering to keep it easy and comfortable.

Then take your mind off your breathing for a moment and just rest. Scan your body and mind and notice any changes you feel since you began. There are no right or wrong answers—just notice whatever you're feeling.

Once you've made a note of any changes you feel, it's time to add some new instructions. You'll begin the same way as before. During the pause while your breath is out of your body, consciously relax any part of your body that feels tense. For example, you might notice during your pause that you're clenching your jaw. If you notice that, just relax your jaw any way you can. When your body signals "time to breathe," let the breath come in all the way and then go out again. Pause with all the breath out of your body. During the pause, find another tense place and relax it. During each pause, find a tense place and consciously relax it. If you find a particularly tense place, feel free to return to it again and again during each pause until you feel it relax. Practice this breathing and conscious relaxing for about two minutes.

Now take your mind off your breathing and rest for a few moments. Scan your body and mind, noticing sensations of wellbeing, clarity, and harmony. Compare how you're feeling now to when you started. If you do the Vibrance-Breath correctly, you will always feel calmer and clearer when you finish. If you don't feel calmer and clearer after a minute or two of practice, it's usually because you're trying too hard to get it right. Don't worry about doing it perfectly—just focus on keeping it easy and comfortable.

The Vibrance-Breath During the Day

I practice for a few minutes in the morning, even though I've felt balanced and harmonious for many years. I think of it as a bit of fine-tuning to help my body remember what the sensations of balance feel like. You can also fine-tune your O-Balance during the day if you get jangled, fatigued, or foggy. Just do a few Vibrance-Breaths at your desk or as you walk around. You can even do a subtle form of the activity in public. I've quietly done my Vibrance-Breaths in all sorts of diverse settings—riding in cabs, giving speeches, appearing on television, and staying alert during meetings.

Once you learn it, you'll have a friend for life.

CHAPTER SIX

Vibrant Connections

The Art of Relationship-Flow

RELATIONSHIPS TAKE ON special importance as we mature. Early in our adult lives, most of us are so bent on establishing ourselves in the world that we don't make time to savor the flow of relationship connection. In our twenties and thirties, we're often willing to sacrifice time spent on relationships so that we can work more, make more money, and attain more power in the world.

In our forties and fifties, we begin to catch glimpses of life's lengthening shadows. We ask ourselves, "What's really important here?" If we're lucky, we wake up and realize that the flow of relationship connection is vitally important. In fact, I believe that waking up to this realization determines whether or not our lives turn out well.

I've counseled thousands of people in their forties and fifties who were struggling with relationship issues. I've had the pleasure of seeing the majority of them discover the sources of their struggles and make the necessary corrections. However, I have also felt the painful, powerless frustration of watching some of them choose to turn their backs on issues they desperately needed to address.

These clinical experiences, as well as relationship challenges in my own life, have led me to a strong conviction: If we do not learn a lesson the first time around, we get one chance after another to repeat it. Unfortunately, each repetition of the lesson comes in a rougher presentation. A number of people have come back to see me—sometimes over a decade later—after choosing to ignore a big relationship lesson from earlier in their lives. Invariably, they'd created a bigger crisis than the one they'd gone through a few years earlier.

It works like this: One winter night in Colorado, I was sound asleep, dreaming of horses. I could hear their hoofbeats thundering across the prairie in my dreams. I snuggled deeper into the warmth of the covers. The hoofbeats grew louder and turned into the rattling and banging of a rickety stagecoach. Then the banging became so loud, I was afraid the stagecoach was going to fall apart. Suddenly I was awake and sitting up in bed.

In real life, somebody was banging on my front door so hard the walls were shaking. I lumbered downstairs to see what was going on. It turned out to be a policeman rapping on my door with his nightstick. He'd come to tell me that a band of marauding yahoos had smashed the window of my car and a number of others parked along my block.

"Sorry I had to bang on your door so hard," he said. "I tried ringing the doorbell, but nobody answered."

That's what happens with our relationship issues. Usually they start softly, like the gentle chime of my doorbell. A spouse may make a simple request, something like, "Honey, would you not watch sports tonight so we can spend some time with the kids?"

Often, though, we don't respond to the gentle chime: "But I'm tired, and this isn't just watching sports, Honey—this is the *play-offs!*"

Bet on it: Next time the knocking will be more insistent. Many of us don't crawl out from under the covers until the policeman's at the door. I know, from staying under the covers too long in a few relationships, that sometimes we don't wake up until the foundation's been cracked irreparably.

Unless you're uncommonly enlightened and incredibly lucky, you will still have some work to do on your relationship issues from midlife onward. It doesn't matter whether you are single, divorced, widowed, in a thriving relationship or a miserable one—there's work to be done. The cost of not doing the work is enormous. When there's a knock at the door, the quick and simple solution is to handle it as soon as possible. If we drown out the knocking, say, by turning up the volume on the television, it usually gets louder until the foundations are rattling. If we hunker down further, perhaps by putting on ear-muffs, we may find ourselves sitting in the middle of a pile of rubble when the pounding's over. That's the big cost of ignoring relationship issues.

That's the cost, but what's the pay-off for waking up and greeting the door-knocker? The pay-off is vibrance, and in order to keep it flowing every day, we must learn to spot and handle disturbances in the flow of relationship. In talking with vibrant people of 50 and older, my colleagues and I found three relationship skills they relied upon to fix disturbances in the flow. Most of them had learned these skills "the hard way."

The three skills:

> Releasing regrets and resentments from the past
> Making key communications
> Planning heartful connections

I had seen the power of these moves, and others like them, in many relationship-therapy sessions. However, I had never realized how strong a role they play in post-midlife vibrance until I took the time to sit down with several hundred vibrant elders. Then it became clear to me what we all need to be doing every day in the area of relationship.

GROWING RELATIONSHIPS

Growing good relationships is like tending a garden. I'm not much of a gardener myself, but I have lived with a masterful one for the past twenty years. My wife, Kathlyn, can make anything grow, from the cactus garden on our deck to the lush jungle outside our bedroom window. Our seldom-used upstairs bathroom has even been transformed into an orchid nursery! She gives her plants a lot of attention every day, and they thrive as a result.

Think of the three skills of vibrant relationships as tending a garden. Like watering a garden, tending a vibrant relationship only takes a little time every day. Of course, if you get behind or have a drought you may have some catch-up work to do.

Regrets and resentments from the past impede the flow of vibrance. Imagine trying to water your garden with one hand while squeezing the hose tightly with your other hand. Holding on tightly to things you feel sad and angry about from the past squeezes the flow down to a trickle. Just let go and you can feel the flow again. It doesn't take long before your plants begin to perk up.

Making key communications opens the flow. Keeping our lips sealed cuts off the flow. Imagine having something you really need to say but being unwilling to say it. That would be like turning the water on full blast but putting your thumb over the end of the hose. Something would eventually have to give. The moment you release the block, you get a surge followed by a steady flow. Relationships work the same way: The moment we express the one thing that needs to be said, we can feel the flow again between us and the other person.

Planning heartful connections keeps the flow going in a positive direction. It's the art of looking for where to spend your time to experience maximum growth. Vibrant people are pro-active people. They look for places to go, people to see, and things to do in order to enjoy the flow of heart-connection on a daily basis.

Each of these skills is an art form that takes practice to master. Let's take a closer look at each of them.

Releasing Regrets and Resentments

Regret and resentment are two different things, but we often experience them as a package. That's because we often leave both of them unfinished in the aftermath of a failed relationship. In our haste to move away from the pain, we store away regret and resentment, only to have them clog the flow of love in subsequent relationships.

Regret is about sadness and loss. It's about losing people and missing out on opportunities. When we're in the grip of regret, we fantasize about a path not taken and our hearts respond with a tug of sadness. Regret takes us roaming through the corridors of the past in an endless search for how things could have been different. A long time ago, one of my clients spoke a poetic phrase about regret: "When I slide into regret, it's like I'm spending eternity re-arranging the deck chairs on the Titanic." We slowly sink while busily trying to get things to turn out differently.

Resentment is a slow-drip leak of anger that's been held in for a long time. It's about holding onto a time in our lives when we were powerless in the face of unfairness and inequality. It contains the bitter aftertaste of a hard-to-swallow feeling of being victimized. When I slip into resentment, my mind dwells on people who got in my way. I think up withering retorts that put them in their place. In my mind, I triumphantly give them their just come-uppance. When I'm in the grip of resentment, I forget temporarily that many of the people I'm zapping have been dead for decades.

The first problem with holding onto regrets and resentments is that it keeps us stuck in the past. Holding onto regret and resentment means we're nowhere near the *now*, the place from which we can give and receive love.

The second problem is that storing up regrets and resentments about people causes us to make up stories about them. We manufacture the stories to justify clinging to the regret and resentment. Instead of acknowledging the real problem—our stubborn refusal to let go of the past—we make up one reason after another to justify holding on. When our minds are clouded by regret and resentment, we think, "Since I'm holding on to so much anger and sadness, there must be some good reason for it." Then, our fertile minds take over and manufacture more reasons.

It's common to hear people say they have "no regrets," but almost everyone has plenty of them. Based on thirty years of helping people with their problems, I think that anyone who says they have "no regrets" is lying and denying. They're usually lying and denying for good reason—usually to protect themselves from the painful task of handling the buried regrets—but even lying for good reason is still lying.

Vibrance comes from acknowledging your regrets but not dwelling on them. Think of a regret as being like people from your past who come up to you on the street. You probably need to say hello, and you may even want to give them a hug, but you certainly don't need to take them home with you. All we need to do is greet them and move on. The same is true for resentments.

The good news: Eventually we get tired of holding onto regrets and resentments. The bad news: Sometimes we don't get tired of it for seventy or eighty years.

A colleague of mine returned from her father's seventy-fifth birthday, fresh with a vivid example of long-held resentment. Her father suffers from Alzheimer's. He often goes for weeks at a time without even recognizing Joan, his wife of fifty years. He was born to wealth but grew richer through his keen business skills. However, his controlling ways with money caused many family problems. The richer he got, the tighter he became. He was notorious for berating his wife about money details— according to him, she always spent too much on groceries, clothing, and things for the children. Tears came to my colleague's eyes when she told me her mother bought everything on sale to avoid being criticized.

At the birthday party, the clan gathered around him to sing "Happy Birthday." Even though he hadn't said a word or recognized anyone during the party, at the end of the song he suddenly blurted out one bitter sentence, "I bet Joan's happy tonight—she's out spending all my money." Then he cackled triumphantly and lapsed back into silence. The accused wife could only stand next to him with her head bowed.

There is supreme irony at work in a situation like that. There he was, safe in his mansion, a millionaire many times over, surrounded by well-wishers and a devoted wife who had spent days organizing the party. Yet, the only thing that mattered was resentment from the past—about something that wasn't even true! This is documentary proof of resentment's holding power. He had long ago lost the ability to control his bowels, but a deeper part of him was still gripping the purse strings.

I don't want to be anything like that when I'm 75, and I'll bet you don't, either. What will keep us from heading in that direction is to get very nimble at releasing our regrets and resentments. Right now. After learning from vibrant elders over the past few years, I make a practice now of releasing regrets and resentments on a daily basis. It's built into our daily Vibrance program, and in a moment I'll show you how to do it simply and quickly.

Making Key Communications

I'm sure you've had the following experience, perhaps many times over. I know I have. There's something you really need to say to another person, but you just can't get yourself to say it. The opportunity to say it comes and goes, and each time you feel worse afterwards because you couldn't work up the courage to speak it. Often it's a simple thing that needs to be said, perhaps

"I felt hurt when you said . . ." or "I don't really want to go to visit your parents." In our research on vibrance, we call them *key communications,* because they open the gate to a deeper flow of intimacy. If they go unsaid, though, they block the flow instantly.

Key communications make a huge difference in how vibrant you feel. Vibrant people know how to say the thing that most needs to be said. They have learned, often the hard way, to take the courageous step of communicating the key thought to the key person. The act of making these key communications not only keeps the flow of relationship connection going but also keeps the flow of vibrance going inside ourselves.

Think of a rapidly flowing stream in which the water is coursing smoothly toward its destination. Then picture what happens if you put a big boulder in the middle. Now, the water has to go around an obstruction to get where it's going. Water doesn't mind—it will cheerfully go around the rock all day. However, we humans *do* mind—if we have to go around an obstruction, we habitually make one of several costly moves.

Sometimes we pull back and lose our enthusiasm for the journey. At other times, we beat on the obstruction until one of us gives in. At all times, though, we take longer to get to our destination than we would if the obstruction were not there.

That's our problem in relationships. If there's a key communication—something that needs to be said—we need to make that communication . . . or else. If we don't, it becomes a boulder that obstructs the flow of connection. Once the boulder's in place, all communication has to go around the obstruction.

Everybody knows, on a conscious or unconscious level, that the obstruction is there (although we can sometimes go for years without acknowledging it clearly).

What Are Key Communications?

The two key communications are facts and feelings. These are the communications that get us in the biggest trouble when we withhold them from the other person.

A fact is something that's happened, a deed we've done, a reality. The flow of relationship connection is disrupted when we withhold a significant fact from another person. Here are examples of facts:

"I stole $30 from petty cash to pay for my daughter's ballet lesson."

"I've been having an affair with the baby sitter."

"I charged a new outfit on the credit card today."

When simple facts like those are hidden, trouble inevitably follows. The hidden fact becomes a lump under the rug that everyone has to walk around.

Feelings such as anger, sadness, fear, and sexual attraction are also key to the flow of relationship connection. One of the most common complaints in relationships is that the other person doesn't share feelings. Here are examples of feelings:

"I still feel angry about the way you treated Doug."

"I'm scared that we're going to run out of money."

"I felt hurt when you forgot our anniversary."

Sometimes the communication is a combination of facts and

feelings. An example of that would be, "I've been thinking a lot about quitting my job and going back to school. But I'm scared you'll get mad at me if I tell you. But I'm more scared of dying inside if I don't go back to school."

Since 1968, when I first began my training as a therapist, I've had the opportunity to witness hundreds of situations in which someone was withholding a key communication—one that made a huge difference. I've always been amazed at the vast amount of energy we spend on dealing with those situations. Perhaps most amazing, I've seen people try to communicate around a huge "boulder" that had been sitting in the living room for years.

In one particularly striking example, a key communication had been withheld for a decade. When it was finally delivered, the key communication boiled down to two simple sentences by a father: "I probably act distant sometimes because I have a whole other family—a wife and two kids—about two hours from here. That's where I go for a couple of days a week, but even when I'm here I think about them a lot."

In this case, matters were complicated even more by the fact that one of the wives knew and one didn't. This strange dynamic had been maintained for most of a decade, until one day the father's heart literally broke under the strain. Fortunately for all concerned, an enlightened surgeon refused to do the bypass until the patient agreed to do the radical emotional surgery of making some long-overdue communications between both families.

Imagine what a huge expenditure of energy it takes to communicate around an obstruction like that! As a teenage daughter of the family put it, "I always knew something was 'off,' but nobody could ever tell me what it was." None of us should have to carry such unnecessary burdens, but the reality is that most of us do. My unspoken key communications have not been so extreme, and I hope yours haven't been, either. However, I've found that even seemingly small obstructions drain energy that could go into more productive activities.

I was well into my thirties before I saw the connection between withheld truths and closeness. What I learned can be stated very simply: If I withhold any significant communication, I will not feel as close to the person I'm withholding it from. If I speak the key communication, I will instantly feel closer to the person.

I came up with a practical definition that made it possible to figure out which communications I really needed to make. A significant communication is anything the other person would have an emotional reaction to hearing. For example, if you think your partner would get angry if you said, "Honey, I'm sleeping with Fred," this would count as a significant communication. If "Honey, I borrowed Fred's lawnmower" would not trigger an emotional reaction, it wouldn't be a significant communication.

I didn't figure out all this until my thirties, when I embarked on a quest to find out why I kept messing up one relationship after another. One of my first big discoveries was that I messed up relationships by not telling the truth about important things. When I shared this discovery with one of my colleagues, he said,

"Funny you hadn't noticed that before!" He had grown up in a family where scrupulous truth-telling was part of the fabric of existence. Early in life he'd learned a simple lesson it had taken me half a lifetime to learn.

My background was utterly the opposite. My family had two main branches—one was an upright bunch who withheld things for moral reasons, while the other bunch lied so habitually that it was just part of the air they breathed. The moral branch, for example, didn't discuss significant things because of principle. As my grandparents put it, "People of quality do not discuss sex or money." The other bunch seemed to lie for less lofty reasons—mostly so they wouldn't get caught doing various outrageous things. However, they almost always managed to get caught in the end, so I figured that lying to them was more like a sport.

This rigorous training in the art of withholding made me a subtle and supple dissembler by the time I arrived at adulthood. Here's an example: My girlfriend might ask me a question such as, "Where were you last night? I called you and didn't get an answer." I would respond with a partial truth, "I didn't get out of my office until after 10 last night." However, I would omit a significant detail, such as "I didn't get out of my office until after 10 because I was necking with a graduate student." As you might suspect, I usually left out the part of the communication that would upset the other person.

Finally, I made a breakthrough observation that would change my life. I realized that whenever I withheld a truth, I pulled back from the other person and created distance. I saw that my acts of withholding eroded closeness. Until I made the significant communication, the distance would grow, becoming a breeding ground for melodramas.

My second big breakthrough came when I realized that I invariably became more critical of other people after I withheld a significant communication from them. For example, if I felt angry but chose to swallow it rather than tell the person, I would start manufacturing criticisms of the person in my mind. If I continued to withhold the anger, I would begin to speak critically of the person to others. Up until then I always assumed I criticized people because they needed it and deserved it. Now I realized that my criticism of them often had little or nothing to do with them—it was about me. I started the whole chain of events by lying to the other person, and then my mind would take the hint and begin to devalue the person by making up things that were wrong with him or her. As you can imagine, this realization was not much fun to entertain.

Although sobering to contemplate at first, these discoveries changed my life radically for the better. In fact, I believe that figuring all this out inspired the quantum jump in maturity that qualified me for my relationship with my wife, Kathlyn. I don't think it was accidental that I met her within a month after I made a deep inner commitment to scrupulous truth-telling. Now, over two decades into a remarkably vibrant relationship, I'm grateful indeed to have become as subtle and supple a discloser as I was a withholder.

Barriers to Disclosing Key Communications

Vibrant people are vibrant partly because they've learned to reveal and release communications that others conceal and hold onto. The ability to reveal and release opens up the flow of connection between people, and this flow enhances vibrance all around. Since it's obviously such a good thing, why isn't it more popular? Why do we often go to such painful lengths to withhold key communications? Why are we so often willing to sacrifice our vibrance for the dubious pleasure of keeping something locked inside?

I think there are two main reasons. The first is that we fear the reaction of others more than we savor the feeling of vibrance. To share a key communication with another person is to risk upsetting that person and in turn ourselves. We would rather feel the familiar state of non-vibrance inside than risk stirring up stronger feelings such as fear, anger, and sadness. Also, we often want to preserve how another person thinks of us, and we fear that sharing key communications will disturb that image. In other words, it often matters more to us what people think of us than how we feel inside.

A moment's consideration would show us the folly of trying to manage how other people think of us. After all, we have absolutely no control over what or how other people think. Why, then, are we so ready and willing to sacrifice our internal sense of well-being in a futile attempt to keep others thinking well of us?

I've thought about that a lot over the past thirty years, and the only answer I could eventually come up with still surprises me. It leads us to the second reason people often conceal key communications. I believe that we, as a species, are intolerant of organic good feeling in all but small doses. We haven't yet grown a nervous system that can handle vibrance for long periods of time. Here's why: Human beings have weathered adversity for hundreds of thousands of years—as a result, we have evolved a nervous system that can tolerate immense amounts of difficulty. As yet, however, we haven't had enough experience with feeling good to develop a capacity for it. A little bit of good feeling goes a long way, and then most of us feel compelled to bring ourselves back down to the familiar state of adversity.

The act of withholding a key communication keeps us in the familiar zone of adversity. Revealing and releasing a key communication takes us out of the familiar into the zone of the unknown. Feeling vibrant for longer and longer periods of time forces us to grow a new nervous system, one that can handle larger doses of good feeling.

If you pay careful attention to good feelings in your body, you will likely notice something very strange going on. If you're like most of us, you can feel really good for a brief period of time—usually measured in seconds or at most minutes—then you will do something to take the edge off the good feeling. You'll eat too much of something, perhaps, or you'll get into a conflict with someone. Before you know it, the good feeling has disappeared.

Before I figured this out, I didn't feel really good for very long at a time. Now I feel great almost all the time. Along the way, I had to notice literally thousands of moments when I "brought myself down" through a cross word, a worried thought, a bumped shin, or too much of a good muffin. I made a psycho-spiritual game out of noticing what I did to take the edge off good feelings that were streaming through my body. After a while, I got so I could feel good for minutes at a time, then hours. At first, I focused on the individual things I did to make myself feel off-center. Then, I took on an even bigger game. My wife and I noticed that the exact same process worked in relationship, too.

We began to notice that we would feel close for a period of time, then something would happen that destroyed the flow of closeness. We started calling this tendency the "Upper Limits Problem." The ways were varied and many: A critical word, a money-hassle, a child's illness, a fenderbender on the new car. As we began to study this problem more closely, we soon realized that *how* we sabotaged our closeness didn't really matter— there was always something. The important thing was *when*. We started paying attention to how much time we had let ourselves enjoy closeness before we torpedoed ourselves with one of our unconscious submarines.

We even stopped assigning blame. We realized that trying to figure out whose fault it was wasted an enormous amount of energy. Blaming was just another way of sabotaging the flow of closeness. We put ourselves on a strict no-blame diet, and this worked miracles on our relationship. Soon we were spending days in the flow of good feeling, even when seemingly adverse things would occur. For example, one of us skidded in a snowstorm and caused $1,000 worth of damage to the other's new car. In the past, this event might have caused a weeks-long disruption in the flow of closeness. Now, though, because we had caught on to the Upper Limits Problem, we looked at each other and asked: Since we've got a bent axle to deal with, would we rather deal with it while feeling great or deal with it while feeling bad? Either way, we were going to be getting an axle fixed, so why not have a great time doing it?

Once you begin to ask these kinds of questions, you've got the Upper Limits Problem on the run.

Planning Heartful Connections

Planning time to connect with people we care about makes a big difference in how vibrant we feel. On the surface it looks like it would be easy: You take a moment to wonder how you could spend your time for the maximum flow of relationship connection. For example, you think, "I love being around Mary. I'll give her a call and see if we can get together." Although it sounds simple and obvious, many of us don't take the few seconds required to make the essential moves. In our research on vibrance, we discovered that the habit of planning heartful connections distinguishes vibrant people from their non-vibrant peers.

How much attention did you give today to planning time with people you love? In other words, how much time did you spend today thinking of things you were going to do that reward you with the greatest flow of relationship connection? When I surveyed people over 50, I found that some of them planned heartful connections every day, but many others never gave a thought to it.

It's important to remember that we're talking about a learned skill, not one you're born with. If you don't know how, it can look as mysterious and difficult as learning a foreign tongue. I strongly urge you to learn how to do it, though, because it has the power to change your life overnight. I know, because I've watched it work miracles with some true "hard cases." One gentleman comes immediately to mind, a retired engineer I spent many hours with. His wife had taken one of our workshops and had made a quantum jump in her vibrance. She wanted him to get the boost she'd received from the program, but he said he wasn't the "workshop type." In fairly good health at 75, he liked to garden, tinker with machinery, and do other solitary activities. When we discussed his relationship connections, he said that he wanted to have more contact with people but felt shy about it. He mentioned in particular that he'd like to spend more time with his only daughter. The way he said it made it sound like she lived in a faraway place, but it turned out she only lived a few miles away.

I asked the obvious question, "Then why don't you spend more time with her?"

"Well," he said, "I spend time with her whenever she calls and asks, but she only calls a couple of times a month."

"How often do you call *her?*" I asked.

He stared at me blankly. He said it had never occurred to him to call her.

I was incredulous. "Not once?"

It turned out he had never once in twenty years initiated a phone call to her. Sometimes his wife would hand him the phone during one of her talks with the daughter, but he had never picked up the phone to call her himself.

"Put yourself in her place for a moment," I said. "If she'd called you hundreds of times but had never received a call from you in twenty years—never heard you say in your own voice that you'd like to spend some time with her—what do you think she might conclude?"

He got the message and picked up the phone to make his call. I was there, so I got to hear the ten-second communication that opened the gate to more vibrance in his life. He simply said "Hi" and "It's Dad" and "I just realized you always call me so I'm calling you this time. Want to have lunch?" When he hung up, his eyes were brighter and his cheeks were flushed. This was only the beginning. Over the next week or two, his vibrance took a quantum leap. It was one of the first times I was able to see closely how much positive energy can come from such a small move.

It's never too late to learn how—you just have to muster the courage to make the first move. In our Vibrance workshops, we start by asking people to make their "top three list" of potential people for heartful connections. Let's do it together right now.

Achieving Vibrance

Here are some questions to get you thinking of who those three people are:

> Who makes your face light up when they walk in the room?
> Whose face lights up when *you* walk into the room?
> Who makes you feel better after you've been around them?
> Who brings a smile to your face and heart when you think of them?

The first three who come to my mind are:

> Kathlyn, my wife
> Kenny, a friend of many years
> David, a friend and colleague since graduate school

Next, ask yourself: What would be the very best way of spending time with each of them so I could feel the maximum flow of connection?

This question requires careful consideration, especially in the lives of busy people. Tune in to each person individually, focusing on the essence of the person and what he or she values, then doing the same for yourself.

With Kathlyn, I came up with an image immediately: a picture of us walking quietly along the beach near our house.

Action step: I decided to invite her to "play hooky" from our normal activities this morning and go for a short walk.

When I tuned in to my friend, Kenny, I had a memory of lunch with him on the deck of a certain restaurant a couple of years ago. When I thought about what was special about that particular time, I realized that it was because our time together was leisurely and uninterrupted. We usually get together at his house, where the flow of connection is influenced by kids, nannies, a dog and cat, parakeets, a couple of assistants, and a chef. Although I have a lot of fun when I'm over there, it's hard to finish a sentence or make a deep connection.

Action step: I decided to zip a fax over to his place, inviting him to try out the new chef at the restaurant we'd lunched at before.

As I tuned in to my old friend, David, I realized that what I most value about our connection is the way we bounce ideas back and forth. I think of talking to him as a white-water run through intellectual rapids. It's always been that way, since the first time we talked nearly thirty years ago. Even though we only see each other a couple of times a year, we can instantly reconnect and resume our wild slam-dance of high-concept banter.

As I tune in, I feel sad that we haven't made the time to connect in probably six months. I scan my calendar to see if I'm going to be in San Diego any time soon. Nope.

Action step: I make a note to call him later and invite him to meet me halfway in L. A. next week when I'm there.

Proactivity and the Essence-Connection

Proactivity—making the first move—is an important aspect of planning heartful connections. Many of us wait until people come to us with a plan and an agenda. Taking a proactive stance has distinct advantages over a passive approach. For one thing, you get to set the tone and the agenda instead of letting others do this for you. Good relationships are built on people sharing the responsibility for the planning.

There is a deeper reason for taking responsibility for planning heartful connections. Think of the two main activities we did earlier:

- Tuning in to people you really want to connect with.
- Tuning in to how you would like to connect with them for maximum flow of heart-energy.

Both of those moves are what I call essence-connections. An essence-connection is when you discover the most sacredly important aspect of someone or something. When you tune in and discover a person who makes you light up inside, you've made an essence-connection. When you tune in and discover an activity that brings forth the greatest flow of heart-energy, you've made an essence-connection.

Ultimately, a vibrant life is created seconds and minutes at a time, by making choices about how we spend our time and with whom. Even a tiny bit of planning greatly enhances your chances of success. By arranging your time so that you make the deepest heart-connections with the most treasured people you know, you take charge of a part of life that becomes more sacred to you as you mature.

A Daily Process: Two Minutes Is All It Takes

In our Vibrance workshops, we teach people a brief process that handles the key relationship issues we've discussed. It works quickly because it's a bodymind process—it engages you as a whole person, not just the mental part of you.

Let's practice the process now. Later in the book, you'll see that it also figures in the Seven-Minute Foundation program.

First, we'll do the "body" part of the process, then we'll add the "mind" part.

1. Sit comfortably where you won't be disturbed for a few minutes.

2. Make two fists and squeeze them as you breathe all the way out. Breathe out "to the very last drop" as you squeeze your fists.

3. When it's time to breathe in, relax your fists and let the breath come in. Breathe all the way in as you continue to relax your fists more and more.

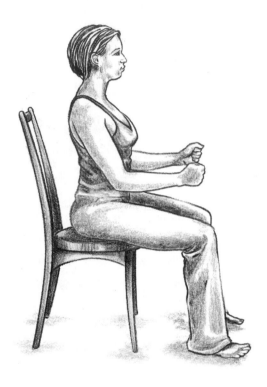

4. When it's time to breathe out, squeeze your fists again as you breathe all the way out. Breathe out all the way, continuing to hold the tension in your fists until you really need to take your next breath.

5. When you need to breathe in, relax your fists completely as the breath rushes in. Keep relaxing your fists and arms and shoulders as you breathe all the way in.

6. Pause for a moment and let's consider what we've done so far.

Metaphorically and physically, we've held a state of tension until we've fully expressed something that needed to be expressed, then we've relaxed as we received the new wave of fresh energy. The full expression of the out-breath enabled us to receive the full in-breath.

Now let's add the concepts of regrets and resentments to the process:

1. Do the same thing you did before—squeeze your fists as you take a full out-breath. As you do, think of anything you regret from your past or present. For example, you might think of a time you hurt someone or told a lie or left someone behind. It's also fine to use a general sense of regret— often a specific regret doesn't come immediately to mind while you're doing the exercise.

2. Think of the regret as you make tight fists and breathe out all the way. As soon as you get to the very end of the out-breath, release your grip at the same time you release thinking about the regret. Let the new in-breath rush in as you relax your fists and let the regret go from your mind. The thought may linger in your mind of its own accord, but have the intention of letting it go even if it floats around for a little while.

3. Do the same thing again on the next out-breath. Think of that same regret or pick another one. Think of it while you squeeze and breathe out. When you breathe in, relax the squeeze and let go of the thought.

4. Keep doing this process for a minute or two. You can use the same regret or pick another one each time.

After a minute or two, pause and rest for a moment.

When you're ready to resume, we'll shift our focus to resentments.

1. Do the same squeeze-and-breathe process on the out-breath, but this time think of something you resent from the past or present.

2. Think of a time someone hurt you or left you behind or told you a lie. If a specific resentment doesn't come to mind, you can use a general sense of resentment.

3. Focus on the resentment through the full out-breath, then release your fists at the same time you release the resentment. Let the breath rush all the way in as you relax.

4. When you're ready, do another round: Squeeze fists, take the out-breath, think of a resentment. Then relax, breathe in, let go.

5. Continue through several more rounds until you've practiced for a minute or two.

When you've finished a few rounds, pause for a moment
to rest.

As you rest, ask yourself two questions:

- Are there any key communications I really need to make
to people? (Remember, key communications are facts
and feelings that would make a difference to the other
person.) If you think of any, jot them down as action steps
for after you finish your program.

- What could I do today for maximum flow of heartful
connections? (Remember, heartful connections are with
people whose faces light up—and who light up your
face—when you walk into the room.) Jot down ideas for
action steps when finish your program.

When you're finished, resume your normal activities.

Enjoying the flow of relationship connection is one of life's joys.
Nobody is born with the skill. We all have to learn it, and sometimes the learning is rough work. However, it's well worth the
time and energy because the prize is priceless. When we
approach the end of our lives, we usually don't regret not work-

ing harder or making more money. We regret the loss of heart connection.

Now, there's a starting place. Take two minutes a day to address this crucial aspect of life.

Get in the habit of doing these three things:

- Release the regrets and resentments from yesterday or a decade ago.
- Speak your key communications into the specific ears that need to hear them.
- Plan heartful connections with people you care about.

One thing to remember: It never gets any harder than this, and it never gets any easier.

CHAPTER SEVEN

Eating for Vibrance

Three Secrets for
Staying Energetic and Slender

≈≈≈≈≈

THIS IS PROBABLY THE FIRST and only time in my writing career that I'll use three exclamation points in a row, but in this case I think they're warranted:

Imagine eating in such a way that you always feel a glow of vibrance inside!

Imagine always feeling a steady, harmonious sense of well-being in the depths of yourself!

Imagine not having to worry about your weight!

If you'd told me ten years ago that these things were possible, I would have thought you were joking. If you'd told me that a way of eating could make me feel harmonious and vital, I would have thought you'd gone around the bend. Now, though, I've enjoyed those benefits for several years and watched many others attain them, too. The good news is that it's possible, and the best news is . . . it's not all that hard.

Like the Zen story says, though, you have to pour out the old tea in the cup before you fill it up with the fresh.

So . . .

I'm going to ask you to do something bold. For the time being, I want you to put aside everything you know about nutrition. That's what I had to do before I could finally open myself to the breakthrough that made vibrant-eating possible.

Begin with a simple question, the same one I had in mind when I began my quest for vibrance. The question is: How can I eat so that I feel vibrant all the time?

BACKGROUND

When I give talks about nutrition, I always begin by saying that I only know one important thing about nutrition—but it's the one thing I'd want to know if I could only know one thing. The one thing I know is this: How to eat so I feel vibrant all the time.

Nutrition is a huge subject. There's a lot to know about it. But if you could only know one thing, wouldn't it be how to feel vibrant all the time? All the rest of knowledge about nutrition may be interesting, but it's not really essential. Eating so you feel great all the time is way beyond interesting—it's life-changing.

Sometimes, in fact, the more knowledge we have about something, the more ridiculous we look if we're not putting that knowledge to work in our lives. Many years ago, I was speaking at a psychology conference at the airport Hilton in San Francisco. It's a popular spot for conferences, and there were several other groups meeting that weekend. As I walked around the hotel I was surprised by the high number of obese people I saw. Finally I found out why.

I got in the elevator to ride up to my room, only to find myself wedged in with half a dozen obese folks. Being in such close proximity gave me the opportunity to read their name-tags: They were all members of an association of dieticians! I started to chuckle, but then I realized the laugh could just as easily be at myself. I knew a lot about a lot of things, but what did I really know? In other words, how much of my knowledge was just gathering dust in my mental attic? How much of it was I really putting to use?

There was a time that I used to feel bad most of the time, simply because of what I ate. When I was in my early twenties, I weighed over three hundred pounds, compared to the 180 or so I weigh now in my fifties. I'm 6'1", so when I weighed three hundred pounds I looked like a sumo wrestler instead of a halfback. I'd been taken to weight specialists galore as a kid, but nothing had ever worked in the long term. Being a smart kid, I also knew everything there was to know about calorie counts and fat grams. I just hadn't been able to put any of this knowledge to use.

When I was 24, I decided to take responsibility for losing the weight, no matter what it required. For a year, I alternated back and forth between eating a fruit-and-vegetable diet and a high-protein diet. When I would get sick of meat and fish, I would eat fruits and vegetables for a couple of weeks. When I started to cringe at the thought of an apple or a piece of broccoli, I would go back to burgers and fish for a while. By the end of the year, I had dropped a hundred pounds. But, oh, that last twenty pounds! I hovered around 200 for years. Occasionally I would get down into the 180s, but then my weight would creep back up over 200 again.

Bill Cosby once observed that when he turned 40, his body stopped producing lean meat. I can relate. In my forties, my weight began creeping up, and as I neared 50 I was pushing 230 pounds. That's when I had my "vibrance" breakthrough. I formed my big question: What would it take to feel vibrant all the time? This question led me to focus on food: How and what could I eat so that I felt vibrant all the time? The question paid off beyond my wildest dreams and resulted in the exciting discoveries I'll soon share with you. It took four years to test and refine our findings on several hundred people. During these four years, I became my own best customer. I'm happy to report that those 50 extra pounds (the weight of ten Manhattan phone books!) are gone now. It took me until my fifties, but I finally figured out how to keep the weight off without dieting.

HOW TO EAT FOR VIBRANCE

It's done by focusing on the *feeling* of vibrance.

I invite you now to let go of all the knowledge stored in your attic about what and how to eat. For the time being, set aside

information about such things as fat grams and protein require-
ments and food-combining. I even ask you to do the unthink-
able: Set aside any prejudice against what one nutritionist called
the "evil white powder," referring not to cocaine but to sugar.
For the time being, let's focus exclusively on the feeling of
vibrance.

Our questions will be: *What* can I eat to feel vibrant all the
time? *How* can I eat to feel vibrant all the time?

Here's what my colleagues and I discovered:

There are no universal vibrance-foods. Your personal
vibrance-foods must be tailored to your body, using a very simple testing procedure you'll learn in this chapter.

While there are no universal vibrance-foods, we discovered
about twenty-five foods that come close. These are foods that
nearly always produced vibrance in the several hundred people
in our study.

There is a simple secret to knowing when to stop eating. If
you master this secret, you can eat practically anything and feel
vibrant.

Focusing on the feeling of vibrance is helpful in losing
weight. Focusing on losing weight is not helpful in learning to
feel vibrant.

Here are the specifics of how to do it.

First, discover your "vibrance-foods." If you put some attention on it, the process of discovering your vibrance-foods will

take a week or so. Once you identify your vibrance-foods, you can move as fast as you want toward vibrance. If you want to take it easy, gradually begin to favor more vibrance-foods in your diet. If you want to feel vibrant right away, eat nothing but vibrance-foods for three days or so.

What Are Vibrance-Foods?

Have you noticed that sometimes you feel sluggish or off-center after you eat? Believe it or not, people have told me they always feel that sluggish, off-center feeling after they eat! They thought it was normal and that everybody felt that way. It's definitely not. It's a symptom of eating something that's not a vibrance-food for you.

By contrast, you may have noticed that sometimes you feel fine after you eat. You feel pleasant sensations in your stomach and intestines, and you feel a calm and energized sense of well-being as you move through your activities. That sensation tells you that you've eaten vibrance-food.

Here's the specific definition of vibrance-food: Any food that is making you feel energetic, clear, and steady an hour after eating it. It's important to draw the one-hour time-distinction. The reason: Many foods are designed to make you feel zippy and cheerful right away. Foods with high doses of sugar, fat, salt, and refined flour fire up your system for a half-hour or so after you eat them. After thirty minutes, those same zippy foods start to make you feel foggy, run-down, and often grouchy. As that sludgy feeling settles in, guess what your body begins to crave. Another zippy food! If this sounds suspiciously like how an addictive drug works, you've caught on to a big secret. It's the key to the spectacular success of the corporate Twinkie-machine. They sell legal addictions.

One of my friends from graduate school went to work for a large company that makes everything from sugar cookies to cigarettes. I talked with him a year later, discovering to my jealous dismay that his job as a beginning research chemist paid over twice what my job as a university professor did. "What do you actually spend your time doing?" I asked. I was secretly hoping they had him torturing lab-rats . . . anything that would make me feel self-righteous about my noble state of poverty.

His eyes shifted guiltily. "I basically spend my time trying to figure out new ways to combine fat and sugar." Noting my puzzled look, he explained, "To make people eat them faster and want more of them."

I thought this over for a moment. "You mean, to make them more addictive."

"You got it," he said.

Suddenly I understood the vast discrepancy between our salaries. It also made sense of the 20 extra pounds that had settled around his middle since I'd seen him last.

Most addictive drugs produce a temporary state of false vibrance. When they wear off, we want to feel that vibrance again, so we go back for more. That's why both cocaine and Coca-Cola are so popular. In fact, I've read that the number-one, -two and -three bestselling products in grocery stores are Coke,

Pepsi, and potato chips. Vibrance is a highly valued state, and if we don't know how to create it by authentic means, we'll pay good money to get it by false means.

Sugar is the undisputed king of the false-vibrance family (at least the legal branch of the family). That doesn't mean it's bad, wrong, sick, or stupid to eat it. It just means we have to be very careful about getting the dose right. Our bodies are not wired yet to handle very much of it.

Here's why: One hundred years ago, Americans ate about a pound of sugar a year. We treated it like a sacrament or a drug, and we used it in small doses, a spoonful a week. Now the average American eats over a hundred pounds of sugar a year! That's a kilo a week, instead of a spoonful a week. For a hundred years, big companies have been hiring smart guys like my chemist friend to find new ways of combining sugar, fat, and flour to saturate our bloodstreams with false-vibrance bombs. They taste great and make us feel great for twenty minutes or so, then the fog sets in, a fog that only clears when we administer another dose. And so it goes. Authentic vibrance-foods don't work like that. When you discover the foods that are genuine vibrance-foods for you, you'll get to keep your feeling of vibrance as an all-day-long steady state.

I'm sure you've found, as I have, that most of the really useful things in life are actually quite simple. Discovering your vibrance-foods is so simple that many audiences chuckle when I tell them how to do it. Like many simple things, though, it took us a lot of painstaking work—with several hundred people and several hundred different foods—to find out how to make it simple.

Discovering your vibrance-foods is a two-step process.

Step one: Eat a food you like.

Step two: Notice your body-sensations 45 to 60 minutes later.

The key is to notice how you feel about an hour after you eat the food. If you feel clear, energetic, and harmonious, you ate a vibrance-food. If you don't, you didn't. It's all about getting that vibrant feeling and keeping it.

Testing yourself an hour or so later is important for another reason. We found, through experimentation, that if you feel vibrant after an hour, you're highly likely to feel vibrant for several more hours after that. That's definitely not true for non-vibrance foods. When you eat something that's a non-vibrance food for you, you won't feel vibrant an hour later and you won't feel vibrant for the next few hours, either.

To give you an example of how this works, let me contrast two very different foods. The first one tests as a vibrance-food for over 90 percent of the people we've researched. The second one tests as a non-vibrance food for over 90 percent of them. In other words, the two foods are at opposite ends of the vibrance-spectrum for most of us.

Our first food will be a large organically grown Fuji apple, providing approximately 100 calories. Nine out of ten people, according to our studies, will feel vibrant an hour after eating a

Fuji apple, especially if it's organically grown. (I'll have more to say on the "organic" issue later.)

Our second food will be two large medjool dates, also totalling approximately 100 calories. Nine out of ten people will not feel vibrant an hour after eating two large medjool dates. There's nothing wrong with dates—it's just that they are so loaded with sugar that they out-score table sugar on the glycemic index (more of this index later, too).

Here's what you would see, if you were watching over our shoulders as we conduct a vibrance-testing session. Ten hungry people each eat a Fuji apple at noon. A second group of ten, also hungry, eats two large medjool dates apiece. At one o'clock, they give themselves a vibrance rating on a 1-10 scale. It measures physical energy, mental clarity, and emotional harmony.

The Fuji group will rate themselves high on the scale, while the medjool group will rate themselves low. If you look at the two groups closely, you wouldn't need a rating-scale to figure out which ones ate a vibrance-food. The date-eaters look a little fatigued. Even though they move more sluggishly, they also look antsy. The apple-eaters look peppy but relaxed.

Everybody's still hungry, though, so we test them on another pair of foods. This time, one group eats a bowl of crispy rice cereal, the kind that entertains you with the famous snapping, crackling sound effects. The second group gets a bowl of buckwheat cereal. Everybody gets the same calorie amount, the same amount of low-fat milk, and a spoonful of fructose on the top. (I'll explain about the fructose later.)

An hour later, the crispy-rice group gives themselves a vibrance rating averaging 4.5 on the 10-point scale. The buckwheat group gives themselves a rating of 8.2. For most of the people we've tested, buckwheat is a vibrance-food. Crispy rice cereal isn't.

Will the same finding apply to you? That's what I want you to find out.

I'm going to give you the benefit of a lot of detailed work by telling you all the foods we found to be high-vibrance foods for most people. I'm also going to tell you the ones we found to be low-vibrance foods for most people. However, I'm going to try to inspire you to do your own experimentation. I know you'll find surprises if you do. You'll very likely discover some foods that you love to eat that don't make you feel good. That may be bad news for you, at least until you learn to eat in an amount that maintains your vibrance. The good news is that you'll probably find some new foods you've never thought of trying . . . foods that make you feel great all day long.

That was certainly my experience. If you'd told me a few years ago that my favorite breakfast would be buckwheat cereal, I might have said, "Buck-*what*?" I don't think I'd ever heard of it. Now I love it, and it makes me feel vibrant. As I write these words, I'm still humming along at peak speed—clear of mind and harmonious of feeling—nearly three hours after eating a steaming bowl of buckwheat with a spoonful of fructose on the top. In fact, I'm even thinking of having it again for lunch.

The Premier Vibrance-Foods

Before I give you our High-Vibrance list of foods, I need to say a word about portions. Practically any food will make you feel non-vibrant if you eat too much of it. Interestingly enough, even non-vibrance foods won't make you feel off-center if you eat a small enough amount. For example, more than two medjool dates makes nine out of ten people we've tested feel non-vibrant an hour later. However, if you nibble half of a medjool date, you probably would not feel sluggish or foggy an hour later.

There's a simple way to figure out how much to eat. We teach it to people in our program, and they've found it uniformly useful:

> Some foods are one-hand foods.
> Others are two-hand foods.

Think of the amount of nuts you could hold in one cupped hand without any of them spilling over. That's a one-hand amount. A small hamburger patty also would fit on the palm of one hand. It might be a little messy, but you could hold it in one cupped hand, so it also qualifies as a one-hand food. It would be hard to hold two hamburger patties side by side in one cupped hand.

If you held out your two hands, cupped together, I could put at least a cup of steamed rice in them without any spilling over, and maybe even two cups. That would be a two-hand amount.

Okay, got the trick?

Here are the punch lines:

- Don't eat more than a one-hand amount of meat or fish. Only one-hand amounts of meat and fish (about five or six ounces after cooking) make people feel vibrant. If ten people eat a typical "restaurant portion" of meat and fish (a half-pound or more), nine of them won't feel vibrant an hour later. We found this to be true even if they are eating a meat or fish that usually tests "vibrant" for them in a smaller, one-hand portion.

- Don't eat more cooked grain than you can hold in two hands. Two-hand portions of cooked grains make people feel vibrant—more doesn't. Eat more than about two cupped hands of grain at a time, and you probably won't feel vibrant later.

Fruits and vegetables are harder to generalize about, because of the variation in their shape, water content, and other factors. Some vegetables are one-hand-amount foods: corn and green peas are examples. We found that people don't feel vital and clear if they eat big portions of corn or peas, along with other vegetables I'll identify shortly. Broccoli is a two-hand food— people feel energetic and balanced an hour after a two-hand portion. Double that amount, though, and most people will feel dull and off-center.

A Word about Organics

I also need to mention the use of organic foods. Some foods we tested only "worked" (i.e., made people feel vibrant) if they were organic. For example, only organic oatmeal rated high on vibrance, while regular supermarket oatmeal rated much lower. The same held true for raisins, grapes, berries, and most apples. My guess is that certain foods are more heavily sprayed with pesticides than others. There is likely something in the residue that detracts from vibrance. (The people being tested did not know whether the given food was organic or not, so their preferences were not likely to have been a factor.)

HIGH-VIBRANCE FOODS

The following foods produced high vibrance-rating in 90 percent of people tested. An asterisk (*) marks a food that only tested "vibrant" if it was organically grown.

FRUIT

Apples*, particularly Fuji, gala, golden delicious, and
  braeburn
Blueberries*
Plums
Cherries*
Nectarines

VEGETABLES

Lightly cooked greens, such as kale, spinach, bok choy,
   collards
Green beans*
Salad greens*
Soybeans (steamed or boiled in the style called
   edamame in Japanese restaurants.)
Bean sprouts

GRAINS

Oatmeal*
Cream of buckwheat
Oat bran*
Kamut
Rye

DAIRY

Kefir and some yogurts
Butter (small amounts)

FISH

Salmon
Halibut
Sea bass
Sardines, drained of oil

MEAT

Lamb

Venison

NUTS

Almonds*

Peanuts*

OILS

Olive

Flax

Bran

Grapeseed

A Good Question

Why do these foods rate high on vibrance? The most useful answer is also the simplest—they rate high because they made people feel vibrant an hour later! The sober, scientific answer is that we don't know for sure. However, our educated guess is that the Glycemic Index plays a role.

The Glycemic Index is a method for measuring the effect of different carbohydrates on the glucose level of your blood. The higher a food rates on the Glycemic Index, the faster it makes your blood sugar go up after you eat it. A high GI food quickly spikes your blood sugar and your insulin response to that sugar. The GI-rating of a food is measured by giving subjects enough of the food to contain 50 grams of carbohydrate, then taking several samples of blood for the next two hours. Fifty grams of carbohydrate is equivalent to three tablespoons of pure glucose (not regular table sugar, which contains a fructose molecule in addition to a glucose molecule). To get 50 grams of carbohydrate from cooked pasta, for example, you would be tested on 200 grams of the pasta (approximately a half-pound, or a "two-hand" portion).

The Glycemic Index has been much in the public awareness over the past few years, but much of what has been written about it is pure bunk. One of my pet peeves is that any number of food-cults and diet-promoters have used the Glycemic Index to justify the theories they advocate. Often, the more extreme the diet, the more inaccurate the information. For example, advocates of one particular diet are emphatic about urging people to avoid carrots. They point to the Glycemic Index as evidence for their radical anti-carrot stance. At first glance you might agree, especially when you see that carrots have a higher GI rating (49) than apples (38). However, if you understand how the GI-value of a food is computed, you would find something entirely different. Carrots only have a small percentage (about 7%) of carbohydrate in them. To get the standardized amount of carbohydrate to test carrots accurately, the researchers require subjects to eat one-and-a-half pounds of carrots. Do you know anybody who sits down to eat that many carrots at a time?

Under normal circumstances, people eat a one-hand portion of carrots as a side-dish, and this amount of carrots would not even have enough carbohydrate to be testable on the Glycemic Index. If the promoters of this diet said, "Don't eat a bucket of carrots at one sitting," I'd be the first to cheer them on for offering this sane advice. By saying, "Don't eat carrots. Period," and especially by using the Glycemic Index to justify the position, they get a raspberry from me.

Details on the GI

Pure glucose is given an arbitrary rating of 100 on the GI, and other foods are compared to this reference number. For example, cantaloupe and pineapple are considered high GI foods, rating at 65 and 66, respectively. Peanuts are a very low GI food (rating: 14), whereas their snack-bag cousin, the corn chip, comes in much higher at 72. Other factors also affect the rating. For example, most bread has a high GI rating because the flour is ground to a powdery fineness and yeast is added to puff it up. The gas bubbles produced by yeast exposes more surface area of the wheat. This makes bread taste better than crunching on a handful of wheat kernels, and it also makes the wheat break down more quickly when it hits your bloodstream. If you ate the same amount of wheat kernels, your blood sugar would register a much lower response than to a slice of bread. Fiber slows the process of breaking down wheat kernels into blood sugar, but when the same wheat kernels are ground into powder, the fiber-advantage disappears.

There is also considerable variation in GI-rating even among members of the same family of foods. I love yellow Finn potatoes, for example, but I don't much care for the big, mealy white pota-toes often served in restaurants. When I saw the Glycemic Index, I finally understood the likely reason for my preference. The waxy, smaller yellow Finns score much lower on the GI than their mealy cousins, and since I'm quite sensitive to blood sugar fluctu-ations, I probably noticed the difference without knowing why.

Now Forget about It

I mention this information about the Glycemic Index as back-ground, not because I want you to focus on the GI. In fact, I want you to do the exact opposite. Forget about the GI and focus exclu-sively on the feeling of vibrance. Choose your diet from interest-ing, tasty foods you like *and* that make you feel vibrant all day.

To help you in this process, here are two more discoveries about vibrant-eating: Vibrance-timing and the V-Spot.

VIBRANCE-TIMING

From our studies, we discovered that you'll feel more vibrant if you pay attention to *when* you eat. The discoveries are very simple, but they make a difference for most people. For certain people, they make a huge difference.

Timing Tip #1

You are much more likely to feel vibrant all day if you do one simple thing: Eat an "early snack," a small amount of protein and carbohydrate within the first half-hour of putting your feet on the floor in the morning. You don't need to eat very much—a half an apple and a spoonful of peanut butter worked for me this morning—but our research indicates that you're more likely to feel vibrant later in the day if you get a little protein and carbohydrate in your body first thing in the morning.

Here are several "early snack" combinations that are popular among our participants:

Half a banana and a handful of almonds
A scoop of protein powder in a small glass of soy milk or
    lowfat milk
Half a bagel with a spoonful of nut butter
Rice cracker with a slice of turkey

I have actually seen this seemingly tiny modification change people's lives. Many people I've worked with initially tell me they can't stand the sight of food in the morning. Invariably, these turn out to be people whose lives change most dramatically when they start eating their "early snack."

Timing Tip #2

Our research also discovered that you enhance your chances of feeling vibrant all day by doing a second simple thing: Within an hour and a half of your "early snack," eat a larger breakfast containing protein and carbohydrate. For example, this morning I put my feet on the floor at 5:45 and had my apple/peanut butter snack around 6:15. Then, after writing for an hour or so, I had a bowl of hot buckwheat cereal cooked in soy milk, sweetened with chunks of apple and a little maple syrup. Then I went back to my writing. Next time I looked at the clock it was two hours later and I still felt vibrant.

Contrast this routine with how my morning went before I discovered how to eat for vibrance. In the old days, I ate nothing until the middle of the morning. Instead, I fueled myself with cup after cup of strong coffee laced with sugar and milk. When the caffeine-buzz wore off and I got hungry, I would usually have a donut or a piece of heavily buttered toast with a couple of spoons of jam. I ran on caffeine and sugar all morning, with a generous splat of fat added on. Somehow I got away with this routine in my twenties and early thirties, but thankfully my body eventually let me know I needed to build a stronger foundation under it. In my thirties, I had a few episodes of dizziness in the late morning. I went to my doctor in a panic, thinking I had a brain tumor or something equally dire. His first question was, "What do you eat for breakfast?" I got the message.

By no means have I become an anti-caffeine or anti-sugar zealot. I still enjoy coffee in small doses, but I no longer use it as a substitute for food. I found that the false-vibrance zing I got from it was fooling my body into believing it was humming when it was really buzzing. As for sugar, I've found that I can handle small amounts now and then, particularly if I remember to eat something more solid at the same time.

Why does eating a small amount of protein and carbohydrate right away in the morning contribute to vibrance? Our theory is that the slow-burning protein and the quick-burning carbohydrate produce a combination of stability and energy in your bloodstream, which you enhance later with a more substantial protein/carbohydrate breakfast. If you skip the early protein/carb snack, the blood-sugar levels may drop so low they have a hard time recovering, even after a substantial breakfast.

Timing Tip #3

A third simple move contributes to all-day vibrance: Eat a small protein/carbohydrate snack about two hours after breakfast and about two hours after lunch. A palmful of almonds and a slice of apple was what I had yesterday afternoon. If you are in the habit of eating a sugar snack or a fat/sugar snack in mid-morning or mid-afternoon, buttress it by adding a small amount of protein. In other words, if you're in the habit of eating chocolate to get a mid-morning buzz, just add a hardboiled egg to give yourself something solid to support the sugar-zing. If you can't get through the afternoon without a donut, no need to go cold turkey—just eat a slice of cold turkey and have your donut for dessert. You're much more likely to feel vibrant if you eat a slow-burning protein along with the fast-burning sugar/fat bomb.

THE VIBRANCE-SPOT

The third secret of Vibrant-Eating is the discovery of a specific sensation that tells you when your body has had exactly enough food. Our participants began calling it the V-Spot, after its sexy cousin below the beltline. The V-Spot tells you reliably when it's time to stop eating. That's a supremely useful thing to know, and a walk down any busy sidewalk in the United States will confirm that a lot of people need to know it.

The V-Spot is easy to locate, but learning to feel it is an art that may take you some practice. After teaching hundreds of people to recognize their V-Spot and use its feedback, I can tell you that almost everyone can learn its secrets if they take the time. Some people "get it" in ten seconds, while others are still struggling to feel it a half-hour later. It's well worth the investment of time, though. Once you get on friendly terms with your V-Spot, you can eat practically anything at any time and still maintain your vibrance.

Locating Your V-Spot

First, let me show you how to locate the V-Spot from the outside. Then, we'll learn how to feel it from within. Learning to feel the actual sensations will give you a lifetime skill you can use every day to enhance your vibrance.

The First V-Spot Experiment: Locating It from the Outside

The best time to locate your V-Spot is when your stomach is moderately empty. If your stomach is too full, you'll have a hard time recognizing the subtle sensations of the V-Spot. If it's too empty, you'll be too hungry to pay close attention. If possible, wait to do the following experiments until you're moderately hungry but not "starving."

1. Trace down your sternum with one of your fingertips until you can feel the bottom of the bone. The bottom of the bone is approximately where your solar-plexus is located.

2. At the bottom of the bone you will probably feel an indented soft spot. If you could see inside your chest, you would see a little piece of cartilage at the bottom of your sternum called the "zyphoid process" (in anatomy, a process is an entity that's fastened at one end but not at the other).

3. Trace with your fingertip about an inch or inch-and-a-half below the bottom of the sternum. Press lightly with your fingertips, exploring gently until you find a place that feels more sensitive than the surrounding area. It feels pleasant if you press, stroke, or tickle it very lightly. If you press harder it won't feel good at all—it will have a "squirrelly" or "funny-bone" sensation.

That's how to locate your V-Spot from the outside. The actual spot is an inch or so into your body (toward your spine) from where your fingertip was pressing.

The useful art of the V-Spot, though, comes from feeling it from the inside. There are two simple ways to do this the first time.

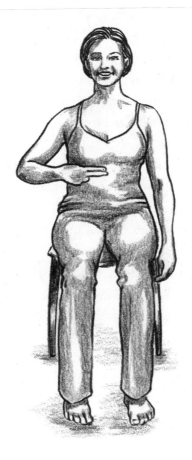

The Second V-Spot Experiment: Feeling It from Within

1. Begin by scanning your chest and stomach with your inner
   awareness. Feel your chest and stomach. Sense the actual

sensations you can feel. Notice them without judging them as good or bad, right or wrong.

2. Now, focus your awareness on the zone at the bottom of your sternum, in the area of your zyphoid process, where your fingertip was just touching.

3. As you focus on that area, swallow several times, about five seconds apart. When you swallow, there will be a subtle fluctuation of sensation in your V-Spot. It's a slight, pleasant tugging sensation just behind and under your zyphoid process.

4. Continue to swallow every now and then, focusing on the sensations, until you can feel the pleasant fluctuation I'm referring to.

5. After a minute or so, pause and take your mind off of our experiment. If you haven't felt the sensation yet, pause and have another go at it later. It doesn't do any good to "try harder" or grind away at it. In fact, the easier you can make it, the faster you'll feel it.

The Third V-Spot Experiment

You'll need five to ten bites of food for your second V-Spot experiment. I recommend preparing bite-size portions of several foods you like before your experiment, so you won't have to stop in the middle to fix more. I'm going to use almonds and a few slices of apple for my version of the experiment. I'll describe what I do, then you can follow along with your own foods.

1. I put an almond in my mouth and chew it slowly. When I'm ready to swallow, I focus my awareness on my V-Spot. I swallow and feel my food as it moves down my throat into the esophagus and toward the V-Spot. At the moment it "hits" the V-Spot, I feel a pleasant wave of sensation. The V-Spot is connected to the opening of the stomach, and the waves of sensation are signalling the transition of the food into the stomach.

2. Place your bite of food in your mouth and chew it up until it's ready to swallow. When you're ready to swallow, focus your awareness on your V-Spot zone. Swallow your food, and use your inner awareness to feel your food travel from your throat down your esophagus toward your V-Spot. Notice that when the food goes through the V-Spot, there's a pleasant wave of sensation.

3. Now, I'll chew up a piece of apple and go through the same procedure again. Please do the same with your second bite. You will likely notice that the sensation (when the food passes the V-Spot) is slightly different this time. It varies from swallow to swallow, and as we will see shortly, this variation is a key to the power of the V-Spot.

4. Let's do the same thing again with our third bite. Focus your awareness on your V-Spot zone as you swallow your third bite. Notice whether you feel as pleasant a sensation as you did with the last swallow of food.

5. Continue to repeat the sequence: Chew a bite, swallow, feel the V-Spot sensations. After swallowing one of your bites, you will notice that the pleasant sensation stops happening. When you swallow a bite and don't feel the pleasant sensations, pause and take your mind off the experiment for a moment. Let's discuss the implications of this simple awareness.

In giving us the V-Spot, nature has equipped us with an exquisitely sensitive mechanism that tells us when and how much to eat. Many people don't stop eating until their stomachs feel full. In hundreds of experimental sessions, we discovered that the pleasant sensations of the V-Spot "turn off" before the stomach feels full. In other words, you will stop getting pleasant sensations from your V-Spot before your stomach sends you signals that it's full.

The big discovery: To feel vibrant, stop eating the moment you stop feeling pleasant sensations from your V-Spot. *If you stop eating the moment the pleasant V-Spot sensations turn off, you always feel vibrant later. If you keep eating until your stomach feels full, you almost never feel vibrant later.*

Your V-Spot won't lie to you like your stomach will. The sensation of "fullness" from your stomach is not a good signal that it's time to stop eating. There's a simple reason for this: The stomach stretches, and if you habitually eat too much, it will stretch so much that it only feels full when it's really stuffed. It will only register fullness when it gets stretched beyond the point it last got stretched to. You don't need to be a gastroenterologist to figure out the consequences of that path.

The Challenge

I predict you will find it challenging to feel your V-Spot sensations in the everyday whirl of life. Even though I'm a thousand times better than when I started a few years ago, I learn a little bit more each day. Dining out is my biggest challenge nowadays. It seems like every week I'm in a situation that causes me to ignore or override my V-Spot sensations. Sometimes I catch myself and remember to pay attention; sometimes I don't.

Two incidents where I really "blew it" come to mind. At a recent gathering, the host had just returned from a business trip to Russia with a huge tin of caviar. There were perhaps ten of us in the room when the caviar was presented, but it turned out that only a few of us were "caviar people." Not only am I a caviar person, I could probably live on it for the foreseeable future. I particularly love the small-grain, fruity-briny type known as Osetra. (Guess which kind he'd brought back.) Here was several hundred dollars worth of my favorite caviar, more than I could possibly eat, absolutely free. All considerations of V-Spot disappeared as the other "caviar people" and I dived ecstatically toward the tin. By the time the carnage was over, I felt like a blimp. A very happy blimp, though.

On another occasion, I was visiting movie-industry friends in Los Angeles. They were going to show clips from some old *noir* films, and I stationed myself on a big couch to watch. There was a bowl of nuts and a platter of homemade brownies right in front of me on the coffee table. I hardly noticed them at first—neither nuts nor brownies appeals to me much. However, the evening took an unexpected turn. One of their neighbors dropped in to watch the clips with us, bringing with him one of his friends. The neighbor was Leonard Nimoy, and the friend he brought was William Shatner. Soon, I found myself flanked by Mr. Spock and Captain Kirk. Now here's the delicious irony: I may be one of the few people on earth who has never seen an episode of Star Trek. I was in a position some of my Trekkie friends would kill for, and I couldn't think of anything to say.

My nerves took over. Suddenly the nuts looked good and the brownies looked transcendent. I'll spare the details, except to say that both of them turned out to be great guys and that Captain Kirk will probably always remember me as the fellow who got chocolate goo all over his hand when I tried to introduce myself.

So, don't expect perfection from yourself. Vibrance-eating is not about doing it right all the time. It's about feeling vibrant, then blowing it, then remembering to eat so you feel vibrant again. Gradually you'll become accustomed, as I did, to feeling vibrant. Your body will gravitate more toward vibrance-foods and less toward the beckoning seductions of the false-vibrance family. One day you'll probably wake up and realize you've been eating vibrance-foods consistently for a long time. You realize you've been feeling great for a long time without even thinking about it. That's what happened for me, and it was well worth the effort to get there.

In the meantime, how about tuning in right now to find out if you are hungry? If you are, treat yourself to a vibrance-food. And notice how good you're still feeling an hour from now.

Enjoy!

CHAPTER EIGHT

Neuro-Gymnastics
The Art of Keeping Your Mind Vibrant

≈≈≈≈≈≈

A VIBRANT MIND is a fine companion to take along with us on our walk through the world. When our minds are nimble, we carry a priceless gift with us wherever we go. It's a gift that keeps on increasing in value—if we take good care of it. In this chapter, we focus on how to nurture and care for that gift so that it continues to shimmer anew each day.

IT'S UP TO US

Many people don't realize that we have the power to fine-tune our minds continuously. In other words, we may inherit a certain configuration of hardware, but it's up to us to make sure we're running the latest software. In this chapter, you'll discover how to update your mind with an innovative, useful, and very playful art: Neuro-Gymnastics. If you take this play seriously, you're likely to be amazed at the enhancement of mental clarity you feel. Even if you're already an Olympic mental gymnast, you may be surprised at the new flips and twists you can learn.

BIG HEADACHE, BIG PAY-OFF

I got the original inspiration for Neuro-Gymnastics from an unusual source: A bad headache. I seldom get headaches, so any time I get one, I know something is going on that I need to pay attention to. Usually the message is simple, along the lines of "Don't drink coffee" or "Don't ski all day in the glaring sun." This one was different—I brought it home with me from a health-food store.

One day my wife asked me if I wanted to go along with her to a huge health-food supermarket that had just opened. She thought it would be fun for me, a confirmed "store-phobic," to try on a new shopping experience. As she shopped, I wandered around, browsing the array of herbs and supplements available for different concerns. Except for taking a multiple vitamin and vitamin C, I don't pay much attention to supplements. I was astonished at the incredible number of products in front of me.

I was particularly drawn to a shelf marked "Mind and Brain." There, I counted over a hundred different products supposed to improve mental function. Since I'm in the "mind-and-brain" business myself, I was piqued by some of the claims made on the packaging. I struck up a conversation with the person in charge, who impressed me not only as a sincere and knowledge-able young man but also a critical thinker as well. I told him I had my doubts about the value of many of these products—to my surprise, he agreed with me. He said, in fact, that most of them were basically worthless.

I asked him why he sold them if they didn't work. He told me that they fulfilled a certain need in their customers. He said that many of his customers were people who were "extremely sensitive to tiny fluctuations in their state of wellness." I jokingly asked him if that was a polite way of saying "obsessive hypochondriacs," but he radiated such an aura of sincerity that my little attempt at humor didn't seem to register. He said that if the products gave people that tiny fluctuation, or even made them think they were getting a tiny fluctuation, then the products had done their job.

"Fair enough," I said, "but are there any that actually work?"

He showed me a couple of bottles. "I don't take any myself, but these are the ones I'd probably take if I had to pick." One was Gingko Biloba, and the other was a combination of various marine algae such as spirulina and chlorella. I was surprised at the high cost of the items, but he assured me the price wasn't out of line. I thanked him and decided to give them a try. I figured that an improvement in my brain function would easily be worth fifty dollars. When I got to my car, I popped the recommended dose of each pill and sat back to await the emergence of the new "me."

Instead, I got a throbbing whopper of a headache.

When I got home, I called my friend, a holistic M.D., to ask if he'd heard of such reactions.

"Sure," he said. "It's not uncommon to have allergic reactions to both of those."

"What should I do?"

He chortled. "I love that question, especially coming from a guy with a Ph.D. from Stanford. If I came to you and said that my wife and I got into an argument every time we sat down to watch TV, what would you tell me to do first?"

"Stop watching TV."

"Right. Get my point?"

I guess I was metaphorically impaired by my headache, because I didn't get the point.

He made it plainer: "STOP TAKING THE PILLS!" I got the point.

MENTAL CLARITY BY NATURAL MEANS

My headache was still pounding away, so I decided to make use of it while I had it. I wondered: What's the message? Immediately, an insight came through—the original curiosity was valid but I'd taken the wrong path. In other words, I was guided to the "Mind and Brain" shelf by a curiosity about how we could make our minds more lively. But then I got off track by thinking that taking a pill was the solution. I needed to find a better way.

I got so excited by the problem that I forgot about my headache. I began to wonder: How could we improve mental clarity by completely natural means? How could we use our own organic resources to improve mind/brain function?

Back in the seventies, I had the opportunity to spend time with Buckminster Fuller, and the most important thing I learned from him was that nature favors simplicity. He always urged his students to ask: What is the simplest possible solution? It suddenly occurred to me that the very simplest solution would be to use our minds in brand-new ways. Right there on the spot I invented a simple experiment I could try out on myself.

To get a baseline, I took note of the sensations in my body and mind. I could still feel the headache, although it was fading into the background, and I felt a slight achy-tired sensation in my shoulders and upper back. My mind was a little foggy, as if I could use a short nap.

Then I began my experiment: I went into the bathroom and did all the things with my left hand that I normally did with my dominant right hand. First, I brushed my teeth with my left hand. Immediately I noticed a difference: My mind was clearer, my body less tired. Then I combed my hair with my left hand. It felt very strange to do it that way, but after I finished, I felt even clearer in my mind. I hadn't planned to shave that day, but I changed my mind and ended the experiment with a (very careful) left-handed shave.

Poof!—no headache, no tiredness. I stood still for a while simply scanning my body and mind. I couldn't feel a trace of any of the unpleasant sensations I'd felt just minutes before. In fact, I felt great.

I knew I was onto something good. Over the new few days, I generated a list of dozens of simple activities—usually taking only a minute or two—which took my mind through new patterns and loops. Then I began conducting experiments with groups of people who were taking workshops at our institute. For example, I would ask one group of twenty people to do an activity that can be done on "auto-pilot," such as counting from one to ten over and over for two minutes. I would ask a comparison group to do one of the Neuro-Gymnastics activities, such as counting backwards from 100 by 7's. It's not possible to do this activity on "auto-pilot" unless you're a math prodigy.

Invariably, the group that did the innovative Neuro-Gymnastics activity would feel more mental clarity, while the "auto-pilot" group would usually feel duller.

The project advanced even more through a happy accident that occurred during one experiment. I was intending to pass out new toothbrushes to two groups, so that I could compare brushing with the dominant hand to brushing with the non-dominant hand. After I got the two groups ready, I realized I'd left the bag of toothbrushes in my car.

On the spot I devised a new experiment: Imaginary toothbrushing. I had one group imagine brushing with the dominant hand for a minute, while the group in the other room imagined brushing with the non-dominant hand.

The group that imagined brushing with the non-dominant hand experienced a significant increase in mental clarity after one minute. The other group had no increase in mental clarity.

Later we repeated the experiment with real toothbrushes, with identical results. The results were striking and opened up a new world of possibilities: Imagined activities could be just as powerful as their real-world counterparts.

Over the course of a year, I refined the activities down to the ones that worked reliably for the largest number of people. In this chapter, I give you the "crème de la crème," the dozen or so best activities we found. You will have the opportunity to do a different activity each day for fourteen days. For full benefit, I recommend that you do them exactly as the instructions specify. For example, if the instructions ask you to do the activity for one minute, do it for the full minute. That way, you'll know that you're opening up the full potential of the activity, and you'll be able to compare your results with people who have gone through our program in person.

FOURTEEN DAYS OF NEURO-GYMNASTICS: THE RESULT YOU'RE LOOKING FOR

Each of these activities is designed to produce a result, one you can actually see and feel. If you do the activity according to the instructions, you should feel an enhancement of mental clarity. Your mind will feel less foggy, tired, or unsettled. Our research indicates that almost everyone gets a positive "blip" of clarity from each of these activities. If it doesn't happen right away, though, please don't worry. Perhaps you didn't do the activity exactly according to the instructions, or perhaps it's just not the right time for you to be doing it. You can always come back and do it again another time. These activities should always be done in the comfort-zone. The only way to do them "wrong" is not to have fun with them.

We begin with the activity I used my very first day.

Day 1

Today, brush your teeth with your non-dominant hand. To help you remember, I recommend using a mnemonic device such as putting a rubber band around the handle of your toothbrush. Otherwise, it's easy to slip back onto "auto-pilot" and use your regular hand.

And remember the most important thing: Have fun!

Day 2

Today, do a new kind of toothbrushing (what one of the program's participants dubbed "brushin' roulette"). Put a coin next to your toothbrush. When it comes time to brush your teeth, flip the coin to determine which hand to use. Designate "heads" for one hand and "tails" for the other. Each time you brush your teeth, you'll literally be in for a surprise.

Day 3

Today, put your clothes on and take them off in a different order than usual. Most people have a sequence that's familiar:

For me it's briefs, T-shirt, shirt, socks, pants. For some reason, I like to put my socks on before I put my pants on, but I notice that my wife usually does it the other way around. Today, though, I changed the order to T-shirt, briefs, pants, socks, shirt.

Let's see what innovations you can come up with!

Day 4

Today we're back to toothbrushing but with a new challenge. When you brush your teeth, combine it with humming a simple tune to yourself.

Tunes that I've used: Beethoven's 'Ode to Joy,' 'Happy Birthday to You,' 'Whistle While You Work,' 'Do-Re-Mi.'

Day 5

Today will be our first Neuro-Gymnastics practice with something most of us do on "auto-pilot" several times a day: Eating. When you eat today, do so with your non-dominant hand. If you habitually use your right hand to hold your fork, switch around. Cut your food with the knife held in your "wrong" hand. Try spooning soup into your mouth with your other hand. You'll likely find that these changes force you to slow down and make eating more mindful. I come from a family of fast eaters, so it's been very useful for me to slow down and learn to eat more mindfully. It's allowed me to savor food more, and I hope it does the same for you.

Enjoy!

Day 6

Today's activity is one that many find addictive. It feels great anytime, but I've found it particularly delicious in the morning.

Several times today, wash your face for at least a minute, alternating between cold and warm water. You don't need to use soap—just the water will do fine.

You can use my technique or invent your own. My way: I have two faucets in the sink I use, so I go back and forth every ten seconds or so. I splash cold water on my face and rub it briskly for ten seconds, then I do the same with warm water. Then back and forth between cold and warm until I feel a brightening of my mind and mood.

It usually takes a minute or so to get the result, but it's never let me down yet.

Day 7

Today I'd like you to do all your grooming and toiletry with your non-dominant hand.

Use your "other" hand for brushing your teeth, combing and brushing your hair, shaving, applying make-up, and anything else you can think of.

Notice carefully when you forget and go on "auto-pilot." What was it that caused you to forget? For example, did you start thinking a chain of thoughts that distracted you? Or did a conversation with someone pull you off-track?

From now on, make it part of the game to notice when and

where and under what circumstances you revert to your habitual patterns.

Day 8

We begin our second week of Neuro-Gymnastics with an activity that looks simple but isn't. In fact, some of the participants in our research say that it's the hardest one to do. These same people, however, rate it one of the most rewarding in enhancing mental clarity.

Today when you eat, put your utensil down after you put the bite in your mouth. Don't pick it up again until you're ready for your next bite.

For example, I had a bowl of granola for breakfast this morning. After each bite, I put my spoon back in the bowl while I chewed and swallowed (and with granola, it can take a while!). On a couple of occasions, I went on "auto-pilot" and held my spoon in my hand while chewing, then I caught myself and put the spoon down.

When I began I felt a little fuzzy, perhaps from being awakened earlier than usual by my cat, Lucy, who was upset by a predawn thunderstorm. After my Neuro-Gymnastics breakfast, though, I felt energized, clear, and ready to get to work.

Day 9

Today do your grooming and self-care routines with either hand, but do something completely different with your feet: Put your weight on one foot, then the other, as you do various activities. If you want to make it even more challenging, balance on one foot, then the other, with your opposite foot off the ground.

For example, I brushed my hair with my non-dominant hand while balancing on my right foot. Then I shifted my weight to my left foot while brushed my teeth with my right hand. You can make up any number of combinations—just keep surprising yourself.

Day 10

Today we do the activity that by definition is the very simplest; It also happens to be the one that people find most challenging.

The French philosopher Blaise Pascal once observed that all the troubles we humans create for ourselves stem from the inability to sit alone in a room for ten minutes doing nothing. After today, you won't be guilty of causing that particular type of trouble again.

Pick a time during the day when you will not be disturbed for ten minutes. When the time comes, sit in a chair and do nothing for ten minutes. That's right: Do absolutely nothing. Don't meditate, don't do breathing exercises, don't consciously think about anything. Just sit and do nothing for ten minutes. When the urge comes up to do something, just notice the urge and go back to doing nothing. If you go on "auto-pilot" and start to do something, stop doing it as soon as you notice you're doing it. Just do nothing.

Day 11

Today we return to one of our favorite Neuro-Gymnastics subjects: Food. One way to break up the routine of daily habit is to use our senses more. Smell is our oldest sense, yet it is one that is overlooked in our civilized world. Today I'd like you to go to extremes with your sense of smell: Each time you eat a bite of food, pause to smell it thoroughly before putting it in your mouth.

As I did this today, I discovered a new world of sensation in the smell of brown rice. Ordinarily, I think of brown rice as a rather boring belly-filler. Today, though, I paid attention to the smell of each bite, and I was richly rewarded with a virtual symphony of scent. Each bite smelled different from the one before! They all had an earthy, nutty smell to them, but they also had subtly different overtones to them. One bite smelled sweet, the next one spicy, another one flowery.

Find out what new worlds you can explore today.

Day 12

Today we re-visit the world of "doing nothing," but we add a new dimension to it that you may find nothing short of miraculous. Pick a time when you won't be disturbed for ten minutes. When the time comes, sit still and close your eyes. For the next ten minutes, just listen to the sounds around you. Don't make a special effort to listen to anything in particular. Just listen.

Let your ears register anything going on around you, wherever you are.

Day 13

Today we link up three different areas of the brain in a way they've never been connected before. Although scientists are still mapping out the territory, many think that our math/logic "machinery" resides in the left hemisphere of the cortex, while our music-making powers reside in the right hemisphere. The part of our brain that organizes movement is in yet another location.

Today's Neuro-Gymnastics puts all those places into play. As you brush your teeth and carry out your other self-care activities, hum softly while counting backwards by 7's from 100. If you get confused or lose track of either humming or counting, start a new tune and start with the next number down from 100. For example, let's say you're humming "Yankee Doodle Dandy" while counting 100, 93, 86, 79. Suddenly you "lose it" and get confused. No problem. Just start again, but this time count backwards by 7's from 99 and begin humming a new tune, perhaps "It's a Small World."

Day 14

For our last formal Neuro-Gymnastics experiment, I'd like you to do something you may want to adopt permanently. Today, change every little routine you can think of.

Here are some starters:

- Eat breakfast out of something different. For example, if you usually eat eggs on a plate, eat them from a bowl today.

- Eat with different utensils. For example, trade your fork and knife in for chopsticks or a spoon today.

- Put your clothes on in a different order.

- Do your toiletry with your non-dominant hand.

- If you usually listen to the radio while you drive, provide your own entertainment, perhaps by singing. (I carry a harmonica in my car for this purpose.)

- Go to work by a different route, even if it takes a little longer.

We'll end with my all-time personal favorite, guaranteed to benefit not only you but others as well.

- At a toll booth, pay the toll for the person behind you. (This one has led to some wonderful experiences. On one occasion, the person took my license plate number, tracked me down, and sent me a box of Godiva chocolates.)

It's up to us to use our minds in ways that keep them alive and well and operating at the speed of life. This is particularly true after 40. At midlife, we begin to get choices presented to us by the day, by the hour, by the minute. The choices are always between innovation and routine. Since life is always changing, it's impossible to try to keep things the same. Refusing to flow with change is hazardous, though, and grows more so as we age.

Neuro-Gymnastics is a powerful antidote to rut-bound routine. It's also enlivening and a lot of fun. I hope you enjoy these activities as much as I have. I also invite you to invent your own, and, if they create noticeable changes in vibrance, please share them with me and others at our website, *www.hendricks.com.*

CHAPTER NINE

Two Daily Vibrance Programs
1. The Seven-Minute Foundation Program
2. The Advanced Program

THE SEVEN-MINUTE
FOUNDATION PROGRAM

Now it's time for us to translate everything we've learned into a few simple, practical moves you can do every day. The Seven-Minute program has been tested and refined over a period of several years. This sequence of activities is the one we've found that produces the maximum amount of vibrance in the shortest amount of time.

Give yourself the gift of doing the Seven-Minute program for a week or so. Take your seven minutes a day and follow the instructions carefully and thoroughly. Then, graduate to the Advanced program for another week or two. By the end of that time, I'm sure you'll have a good sense of whether vibrance is for you.

As I mentioned earlier in the book, the most common mistake is that people stop doing the program because it feels so good. They start to feel more vibrant immediately, and the feeling of increased well-being triggers their "Upper Limits" thermostat setting. A little voice most of us have in our minds kicks in and says, "You don't deserve to feel this good," and—lo and behold—next thing you know it's been a few days since you've remembered to do the program. Be aware of this tendency, and don't let anything stop you for those first couple of weeks.

Now, set aside seven minutes and move through the three steps of the program.

Step One: Vibrance-Flexing

The biggest secret to staying vibrant all day is learning how to keep your spine flexible. Nature has designed your spine to move in an ideal way—with the Vibrance-Flex you re-create this ideal movement for a few minutes each day. Gradually, your bodymind will remember the movement and begin to do it spontaneously. Until it becomes second nature, a few minutes of daily practice is the place to begin.

Begin with the seated Vibrance-Flex. (If you need a refresher of the instructions, look on pages 83–86.)

After warming up your body with a few cycles of the seated V-Flex, add your breathing in coordination with your movement. Breathe in fully as you arch the small of your back, and breathe out fully as you flatten the small of the back. (If you'd like to refresh your memory of the complete instructions, they're found on pages 86–89.)

Step Two: Vibrance-Breathing

After a few cycles of the seated V-Flex and breathing, take a couple of minutes to balance your oxygen and CO_2 levels by doing the Vibrance-Breath (full instructions on pages 113–15).

Step Three: Relationship-Flow

Devote two minutes to getting your relationships off to a fresh start. Do the relationship process detailed on pages 143–47.

In just a few minutes, you've accomplished several remarkable things: You've flexed your spine to get your vital energy flowing. You've filled your body with full, deep breaths that put your system into harmony. You've let go of unfinished relationship business from the past and planned heartful connections that will bring you a satisfying flow of relationship contact in the present.

Enjoy!

THE ADVANCED PROGRAM

The Advanced program is built on the solid foundation of the Seven-Minute program. The Advanced program contains some powerful additions to the first two steps of the Seven-Minute program. You've been doing a basic Vibrance-Flex and Vibrance-Breathing activity in the Seven-Minute program. In the Advanced, you do the full series of Vibrance-Flex and Vibrance-Breathing activities. The Third Step (Relationship-Flow) stays the same as in the Seven-Minute program.

Chances are, you'll feel a bigger surge of vibrance the first day you move up to the Advanced program. If you don't, go back through the instructions for the Foundation program, taking care to do them for the specified length of time. The most common mistake people make with the Advanced program is to "cut corners" with the Foundation program it's built upon. In their eagerness to get to the Advanced activities, they skip over the basics. That's a mistake. If you shave time off the activities in the Seven-Minute program, you won't build that strong foundation of vibrance that we're trying to generate in your bodymind every day.

Step One: Vibrance-Flexing

Your first step begins with the seated V-Flex. (Instructions on pages 83–86.)

Then, move on to the standing V-Flex. After a minute or two of this exercise, pause and rest with your arms at your sides. When you're ready, add the following advanced instructions.

1. While standing, jiggle your right hand gently, keeping the wrist joint open and free. As you jiggle the hand and wrist,

also relax your finger-joints so that they jiggle freely along with your hand and wrist. Add your elbow joint and shoulder joint to the play. Jiggle them gently along with your wrist and hand and fingers. Continue for thirty seconds or so, then pause to rest.

2. Compare the sensations in your right arm with the sensations in your left. Notice the difference between the arm you've been jiggling and the other one. You may feel a flowing, tingling sensation in the one you've been jiggling. Now, shift to your left hand. Begin jiggling it gently, letting the wrist be open and free. Relax your fingers so they jiggle loosely along with your hand and wrist. Let your elbow joint and shoulder joint begin to join the play. Keep the jiggling easy and gentle and playful. Continue for thirty seconds or so, then pause to rest.

3. Shift your attention to your legs. Take your weight off your right leg. You can touch the wall to balance yourself if you need to.

4. Jiggle your right ankle. Most people find this more challenging than jiggling a wrist or shoulder. There's usually more tension in the lower parts of our body. Do the best you can to let your foot and toes be loose as you jiggle your ankle. Remember to stay in the comfort zone, gentle and easy.

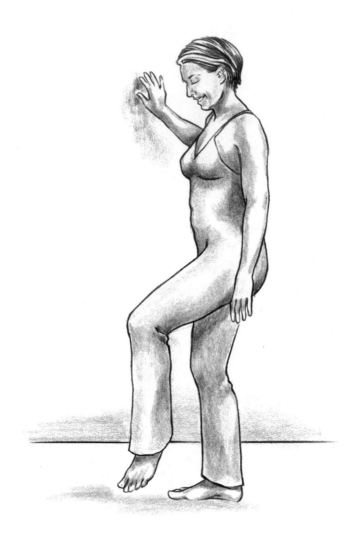

Include your knee and hip joint in the play. Jiggle them gently and playfully along with your ankle and foot.

5. After 30 seconds or so, shift to your other leg. Jiggle your left ankle, then include your foot, toes, knee, and hip joint. Keep the movement playful and gentle.

6. Now, jiggle your right hand and arm as you continue jiggling your left leg. Let the various joints communicate with each other. For example, get the jiggling of your right wrist into harmony with your left ankle. Play with different variations of communication between various joints. After you've done this for 30 seconds or so, switch to the opposite sides. Jiggle your left hand and arm at the same time you're jiggling your right ankle and leg. Strike up "conversations" between the various joints. Keep the movement gentle and playful.

7. To finish, put both of your feet back on the floor. Randomly jiggle all the joints of your arms and legs. Make the movements as playful as you possibly can. Make them smaller or larger, faster or slower. Play with variations. For example, jiggle your left arm slowly as you jiggle your right leg fast. Surprise yourself with unusual innovations. Continue as long as you want, then pause and rest.

Step Two: Vibrance-Breathing

In the Advanced program, you begin with the same breathing activities you already learned in the Foundation practice. Then you add an advanced breathing activity that is done lying down. (If necessary, refresh your memory with the instructions found on pages 113–15.) After you do several minutes of the seated activities, lie down for the final two advanced breathing processes. If possible, do the activities on a firm, comfortable surface. A carpeted floor or a gym mat is ideal.

1. Rest your arms on the floor at your sides. Bend your knees and bring your feet up so they're flat on the floor.

2. Arch and flatten the small of your back. Arch away from the floor, then flatten the back into the floor. Make it a gentle, rolling movement. Relax your neck so that the movement of arching and flattening your back tugs your head slightly up and down. Do this movement slowly and gently for a few cycles, then pause and rest.

3. Start the movement again, this time coordinating your breathing with it. Bring in a full, deep belly-breath as you arch the small of your back, then breathe out slowly and deeply as you flatten the small of your back. Let your belly round fully when you breathe in, and then let it flatten completely as you breathe out. Move gently and slowly, focusing

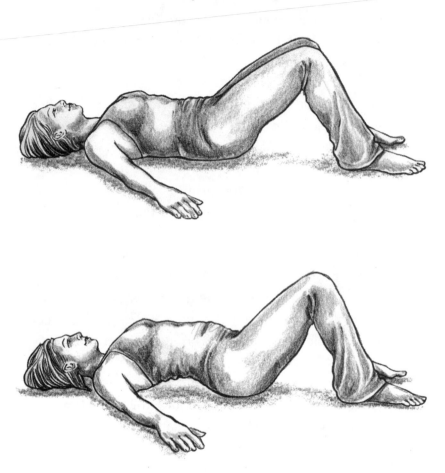

your attention on the sensations of the breath coming in all the way and then emptying all the way out. Practice for a minute or two, then pause to rest. When you pause to rest, stretch your legs out flat on the floor to give them a break.

4. Bend your knees again and slide your feet up so they're flat on the floor. Stretch your arms straight out from your shoulders in a T-position.

5. Roll one arm up the floor as the other arm rolls down. When you've rolled all the way in one direction, make a smooth transition to rolling back the other way. Keep both arms moving simultaneously. Make sure you roll the arms—don't slide them up the floor. You want to roll the shoulder joint through its full range of motion in both directions.

6. When you've got your arm movements rolling smoothly up and down, add your legs in the following way: Roll your knees over toward the side where your arm is rolling down the floor. Then roll them back to the other side when your arm starts rolling back up the floor.

7. When you've got your arms and legs moving smoothly together, complete the movement by letting your head roll to look away from the direction your knees are dropping. Another way to say this is to roll your head in the direction of the arm that's rolling up the floor. Coordinate these movements together until they feel smooth and natural.

8. When it feels smooth and natural, add your breathing in the following way: Take your in-breath as your knees drop to the side, then start your out-breath as they come back up toward

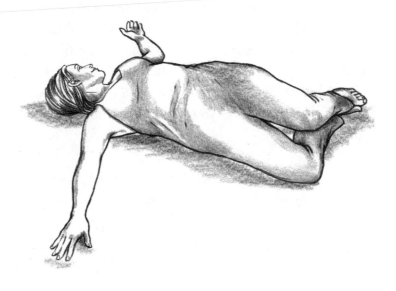

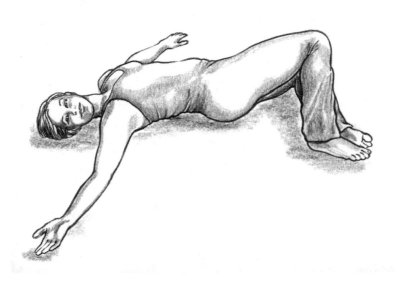

the midline. Then take your next in-breath as they drop to the other side. Make the movement very slow, so that you can breathe slowly and deeply in harmony with the movement. Feel how the stretch opens the front of your body for a full in-breath. Feel how your breath can move the whole front of your torso, from your collarbones down into your groin.

9. Enjoy this movement for a couple of minutes, keeping it slow and gentle. When you feel ready to finish, stretch your legs out flat and rest your arms at your sides. Rest for a few moments before you resume your normal activities.

Step Three: Relationship-Flow

Carry out the relationship-flow activity exactly as before (instructions on pages 143–47).

A VIBRANT FAREWELL

It has been more than a pleasure and an honor to share this work with you—it's the fulfillment of my life purpose. Many years ago, I formed the guiding purpose of my life: to expand in vitality, love, and creativity every day as I inspire others to do the same. The development of the Vibrance program has been in every way the most satisfying expression of this life purpose that I could have ever dreamed of.

Certainly my personal experience has been satisfying. I use the practices myself to feel better than I ever imagined, and they've been essential in helping me expand in vitality, love, and creativity. However, the satisfaction of feeling my own vibrance pales in comparison to the heartfelt exhilaration of watching hundreds of people every year discover their natural vitality, clarity, and harmony. I've been blessed for years now to live in a constant state of awe, surprise, and wonder at how magnificent people can be when they allow themselves to be.

Now you know everything I do about how to enjoy a vibrant life—here's to the daily flowering of your magnificence!

Using the Vibrance Program in Conjunction with the New Generation of Medical Anti-aging Treatments
by Darren Clair, M.D.

The Vibrance program described in this book is a breakthrough paradigm for those who want to stay young in mind, body, and spirit. Vibrance is an active process, a dedication to looking at each day as a new experience and a new opportunity to learn and grow. At present, the field of medicine is also developing a new generation of anti-aging treatments which can substantially enhance Vibrance. When used in combination with the mind-body approach of the Vibrance program, a veritable "fountain of youth" is finally within reach.

It all starts with flexibility. When we work on ourselves to remain flexible, we not only survive but prosper. The reason flexibility is so important is that it allows us to deal more effectively with the stresses of life. We live in a world where the only certainty is change. What sets humankind apart is our ability to find new solutions when the old ones aren't working anymore—in other words, flexibility. The magic of Dr. Hendricks' program is that he shows us exactly how we can keep our flexibility increasing in every possible way.

Before starting the Vibrance program there were more than a few mornings when I woke up stiff and still tired, feeling old. This didn't happen overnight. I got to that point from a culmination of never-ending stresses at every level of my being. To generalize to our communal experience, when cells can't deal with the stress of damage to the DNA, those cells are no longer productive. They cannot produce the necessary proteins or they die or become cancerous and thereby become added stress in themselves. When organs are inactive they, too, age. Inactivity leads to bone deterioration and weak, stiff muscles and both of these lead to osteoporosis. Inflexibility leads to the dowager's hump and the lens stiffness of presbyopia. The inflexibility due to overstretching of heart muscle fibers of congestive heart disease leads to heart failure when the heart can no longer adequately contract and pump the blood. Inactivity of the mind leads to memory loss and contributes to dementia. The inflexibility of oft-repeated opinions leads to dogma and closed mindedness and neither of these helps us deal with an ever-changing world. Clearly, we want to avoid inflexibility at all costs unless it truly threatens our safety.

Using the tools that Dr. Hendricks describes in this book will have a remarkable effect on your life. Because of the power of the mind-body connection you will feel, act, think, look, and be more youthful if you make the conscious decision to incorporate these exercises and habits into your daily routine. This is the most important step to take, and I urge you to take it now. You must first commit to flexibility and activity. Once you have made this step there are other powerful tools at your disposal to maximize your Vibrance. Medical science in the twenty-first century has given us a better understanding of the physical reasons we age and lose our Vibrance. We can now use that understanding to slow aging and enhance Vibrance.

I know from personal experience and that of my patients' that a synergy occurs when the work (play) that Dr. Hendricks describes in this book and the new medical breakthroughs combine so that the results are even greater than might be expected or hoped for. After a few weeks on hormone supplementation I noted improved energy levels especially in the late afternoon and an improved mood experience as an ability to deal with problems with a more constructive, "this is fixable" attitude. Since starting the Vibrance breathing and stretching exercises in the morning I have recently noticed that I am singing to myself in the morning and (to my daughters' dismay) to them as well.

What happens to the Vibrance we can usually see in our childhood photographs? Life happens. Stress is a fact of life from the moment of conception. And whereas some people feel that stress is bad, it is not the stress that is the problem. The real problem is how we react to the stress. Stress can help us grow stronger physically and mentally. As Nietzsche put it, "If it doesn't kill you, it will make you stronger." We have within us an amazing multi-level, overlapping array of repair systems to deal with practically any stress we may face. If we are able to effectively handle the stress because the necessary DNA repair systems, hormones, immune system, quietness of mind, or social support system are not only present but also fully functional, then instead of leading to decline, the stress can lead to further growth and flexibility—to more Vibrance.

When our support systems and repair systems are down, however, stress leads to irreparable damage. When the damage is allowed to continue we physically age. Aging is first and foremost the overwhelming of our support systems by chronic multi-faceted stress. To slow the aging process and maximize our Vibrance we must maintain our repair systems in optimum shape.

As products of an incredible evolutionary process we have within us a multi-level, interacting, redundant reparative and restorative system that is built into our DNA—the molecular blueprint involved in almost every aspect of ourselves.

As an example of this wonderful failsafe system, the DNA itself is present in duplicate in every cell in the body. What is more, the genetic plan for many of the important proteins is encoded multiple times in the DNA. On top of these insurance policies the cell contains enzyme repair systems that correct any damage to the DNA. All these measures are present within each cell at the nuclear level to ensure that when the DNA is copied it is copied exactly so that the cell remains healthy and when it divides the resulting cells are perfect.

At the cellular level there is another level of integrated system repair. One example of this is the coating of each cell with protein markers that identify each cell as a healthy part of the person so that foreign-invader organisms, toxins, or cancerous cells are eliminated by the immune systems' white blood cells.

As an individual we are programmed to take our stresses in digestible doses. We eat meals and take a break from eating to allow proper digestion. We sleep at night. We stay home and rest when we are sick because we have temporarily (hopefully) overwhelmed our safeguards against infection. This can be due to playing outside without a coat or perhaps dealing with the emotional stress of relationships. While writing this I am nursing a cold brought on by the stress of looking at childhood abandonment issues. What my body is telling me is to stop and take the time I need to heal this old hurt.

As a society we organize ourselves into families and communities to nurture and protect individuals within the group for the best interests, not only of the individual, but more importantly, of the species.

Why do repair systems break down? What went wrong with this exquisite example of evolutionary genius? I believe it is not a matter of what went wrong so much as what is going so right. Mankind has been around for millions of years but it has only been within the last 100 years that the life expectancy has increased from about forty to close to eighty. That is an incredible jump in a brief period of time. The whole human organism evolved with a forty-year life span in mind. Our life cycle is based on this. It's why we peak in our twenties and early thirties. Our repair systems are also geared to peak in our twenties and thirties. That is when we are fertile and have children, when we are most healthy, and after that period, we start aging. After we have contributed to the continuation of the species we are a burden to the species because we no longer producing young. We are also consuming nutrients that in a hunter-gatherer society would go to younger, fertile individuals.

We have evolved as hunter-gatherers on physical level. With modern medicine we have essentially ended evolution on this level. Evolution now continues, though, on mental and spiritual planes. This being the case it is useful for us to live more than forty years. After we are no longer burdened by the necessity of caring for the young we can spend more of our time exploring our inner world. And as we live to see several generations grow, we can get a better appreciation of the importance of the values we consider more evolved—empathy, compassion, and truthfulness.

All of our systems, however, are programmed to the hunter-gatherer lifespan timetable. Modern medicine has a good understanding of some of the changes that occur in our bodies after the age of forty—leading to what we recognize as aging. First and foremost is the decline in hormone levels. Hormones are messengers, molecules that are produced in different organs in the body which influence the growth and behavior of cells in other parts of the body. Insulin, for example, produced in the pancreas, tells my fat cells throughout my body to store excess calories in the form of fat. There are several other hormones produced in our bodies and the production of most of them declines slowly after peaking in our thirties. As these hormones are produced less they are present in lower levels in the blood and target tissues. Just as juvenile diabetics make no insulin and therefore cannot store sugar and as a result have high blood-sugar levels, the decreased levels of other hormones result in decreased activity in the target tissues.

What's most exciting is the finding that by supplementing the amount of hormones in the body we can affect the activity of the target tissues. When the hormones are supplemented to the levels of a thirty-year-old, the target cells act as if they were thirty, and as a result, we slow the aging process. A demonstration of this is the effect of female hormone replacement therapy—estrogen and progesterone—on bones where these hormones can stop and even reverse osteoporosis, once thought to be irreversible.

Growth hormone and DHEA are two important hormones along with the sex hormones in the life enhancement armamentarium. Growth hormone, or HGH, is an important regulator of many processes throughout the body, besides the part it plays in our growth in height as children. By supplementing this hormone to optimal levels, we have seen dramatic improvements in many indices of aging—decreased body fat, especially the "spare tire," increased muscle mass, improved energy and mood, improvements in memory, increased bone density, strengthening of the immune system, and much more. DHEA has many of the same effects on the patient's physique but to a lesser degree.

Here again we see the importance of synergy—when all the hormones are brought up to optimal levels the improvements are greater than the sum of the individual hormone's enhancing effects. In some ways its like the old car that you decide not to trade in but instead put a little money into. You start by replacing the carburetor and notice a little improvement. Sometimes, however, you find it is not until you have replaced the whole engine that it really seems to drive more smoothly. In addition, the more hormone levels that are optimized, the lower the dosage of each of the hormones that is necessary to get the desired effect.

How can you maximize your Vibrance? My experience has shown, and the experience of my patients has confirmed, that it's best done by a synergy of mind-body activities and the leading-edge medical solutions now available. By combining the mind-body exercises that Dr. Hendricks describes with the advancements of modern medicine, you now can greatly increase your vitality and your ability to enjoy your life.

INDEX

Index

Index

Index